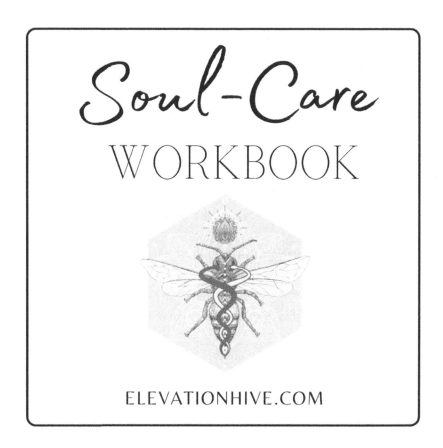

Soul-Care
WORKBOOK

ELEVATIONHIVE.COM

Amanda Lux, BCPP

Published by: Elevation Hive School of Energy Medicine

For permissions or to obtain copies of this book please contact: Be@Elevationhive.com

All photos of Amanda Lux are by Dzhan Wiley at DzhanWiley.com

For free resources, information, access to the accompanying online course, and for fillable PDF worksheets from this book go to:

Elevationhive.com/soul-care-book

Important Disclaimer: The information contained in this book is not intended to diagnose or prescribe. The contents are intended to educate, inspire and support you on your journey.

Please consult your healthcare provider. Any use of the information contained in this book is at the discretion and sole responsibility of the reader. The author bears no responsibility.

ISBN: 978-1-7351232-0-2

Dedication

This book is dedicated to the sacred lineage of this work that began with Dr. Randolph Stone,

the ultimate seeker, and visionary who founded Polarity Therapy.

And to the incredible teachers at the Life Energy Institute who brought it to me;

Gary Strauss, Tracy Griffiths, Dina Fraboni, and Lynn Dennison.

Thank you for every rite of passage, word of wisdom, and for the authenticity and integrity of your transmissions.

Acknowledgments

A huge thanks to Kelly Watkins for your inspiration, collaboration,

and friendship; to Lisa Cosmillo for the edits;

to Dzhan Wiley for the incredible photos and a life of shared poetry;

to Karuna for helping me access my dreams;

and to my family for being awesome.

Exclusive Reader Offer!

Save $97 and get the online course for FREE

Elevationhive.com/soul-care-book

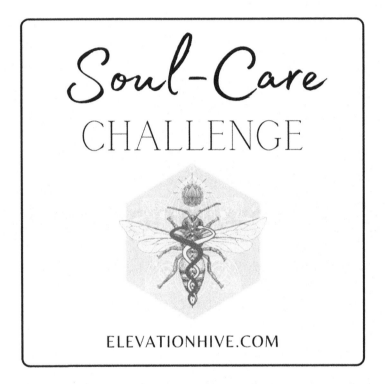

Join the community & follow us!

TABLE OF CONTENTS

SECTION ONE: INTRODCUTION

CHAPTER ONE: WHAT IS SOUL-CARE?

Soul-care is a multidimensional version of self-care. It is about tending to your physical, emotional, and mental bodies, as well as your rituals, desires, dreams, essence, and energy. It's about devotion to the self and the inner sanctity of your sacred beingness. It's about tending your relationship to the Mother, this planet that holds, nourishes, and provides for you.

Most of all, Soul-Care is about hunkering down, digging in, gently, compassionately turning towards and within so that you may develop a practice of listening and tuning in to your energy and, therefore, your whole being. This workbook was created to educate and support you in real and practical ways to understand energy medicine through the lens of your chakra system elementally. In the context of this workbook, Soul-Care is where the rubber meets the road, spiritually speaking. Beyond caring for our minds and bodies, this is about tending to your subtle body holistically.

Your subtle body makes up the 99% of you that comes from the mystery. It is the vast aspect of you that is creating your experience. It is underneath the thoughts and vibrations that give rise to your pains and pleasures, your illnesses, and your accomplishments.

We have access to all the wisdom of the ages at our fingertips. We can read all the books and agree with all the inspirational memes that scroll across our feed, but until we weave the concepts into our lives, they remain ephemeral, intellectual, two dimensional.

This workbook aims to distill the fluff into an actionable, doable, fun, life-altering, healing, balancing practice. A practice that you get to cultivate along the way.

Who is this book for?

This book was originally created for empaths, sensitives and healing arts professionals looking for tools and resources to both moderate their sensitivities and cultivate them. Creating a daily practice of tuning in to one's energy is supportive for anyone who endeavors to show up for others in a therapeutic context. Whether you are a bodyworker, energy worker, therapist, student, educator, yoga teacher, or seeker looking for tools and practices to support or develop your sensitivities, this book is for you. It is also for anyone with the courage and willingness to step on the path.

How I came to this work (My 'Why")

Much of what I have learned about self-care for the soul has come from working one-on-one with private clients for more than 17 years. I have run a private practice as a Polarity, Craniosacral, and Massage Therapist, Intuitive Energy Worker, DreamWorker, BodyMind Bridge Hypnotherapist and Transformational Life Coach. This life path has provided me with the incredible opportunity to facilitate somewhere in the vicinity of ten thousand sessions. They say when you do something ten-thousand times, you become an expert. And while this may be true in some ways, I also tend to think I am just a slow learner. Beyond a firsthand appreciation for the old saying, 'the more you know, the more you know you don't know', I think the one thing I can claim to have gathered from this experience is a love for listening.

Working with so many amazing clients has allowed me the opportunity to cultivate a fascination for the subtleties of how energy expresses, and an appreciation for the nuance of how it is communicated through each of us uniquely. I have learned to witness reverently- to reflect upon and with each client what has worked and not worked in their lives physically, emotionally and spiritually.

I have been involved in countless conversations, both spoken and unspoken, which have taught me so much about what it means to be human in a body full of struggles and aspirations, traumas, and dreams, all wound together into layers of tissue and emotion.

Over the years, I have learned to palpate the soul through muscle, sinew, and bone. I've learned to hear the silent ways that grief cries out when it is unexpressed- to feel in my own body, how other people's pain or disconnection shapes the postures they take and informs the gestures they make, and to recognize the accumulation of experiences that need digesting, witnessing, transmuting or honoring.

But to hold space for other people's soul-care and personal tending, I have had to cultivate a deep relationship with my own. As an empath, healing arts practitioner and teacher of energy medicine, my sensitivities are my greatest assets. But only as long as I take impeccable care of myself. When I forget to use the tools that help me most, then my sensitivities feel like a huge burden. They turn into something I have to overcome. At times, it has taken everything I had to focus on remembering how to do this healing-through-radical self-love-thing. But with regular practice, persistence, and devotion to tending to my own energy system, I have cultivated a deep appreciation for my sensitivities. I have found tremendous freedom, ease, and joy in knowing myself that I wouldn't trade for anything. I have spent so much time and energy trying to figure out what I need to stay open and how to get the mix right, often by doing it wrong. ***But that is the nature of Soul-Care.***

Being self-aware and tending to our growth multidimensionally allows us to be more authentically ourselves, which is the only way we can really show up for others sustainably. It takes work but over time it becomes second nature and life gets more amusing, the messages get clearer and easier to read, and the whole trip just gets more beautiful and interesting. This keeps me on the path. Ever curious of where it will take me next.

Along the way, I have continually heard a call to connect with others through sharing, teaching and gathering like minds for healing because I feel it is essential that we do some of this work in community. It is not easy but oh-so much easier when we find our tribe and endeavor to uplift one another. It is this dream of community that has fueled my desire to start the Elevation Hive School of Energy Medicine; a place for like-minds to connect, learn and grow. It takes humility and grit to transform our wounds into wisdom, and this only comes from regularly engaging with our energy, emotions, and truth through practice.

It is my sincere wish that this book speaks to the place in you that is ever returning to the realization that you are worth the effort it takes to do this for yourself. May this book and our other offerings provide inspiration, encouragement and support along the way as you cultivate the landscape of your soul. Many blessings on your Soul-Care journey!

How to use this book

This book is intended to offer practical ways to learn how to work with your energy system. Most of the exercises are based in Polarity Therapy but all of them were chosen because they are accessible, adaptable and do not require a huge investment of time or money.

You will find simple ways to listen to and honor yourself throughout your everyday life. Each prompt has come from personal experience. These practices have supported me throughout my life and have benefitted my clients and students as well.

There is an online course that accompanies this workbook. Learn more about the course and view all other links and resources at elevationhive.com/soul-care-book This elemental journey is greatly enhanced when it is experienced as an interactive process where you can receive support and accountability. But it is also something you can do on your own.

This book was set up originally to be a 33-day consecutive journey, however, the only way you can get this wrong is if you berate yourself for falling "behind." *Which is why you are invited and encouraged to be on your own timeline.*

If it is helpful for you to have the daily reminders to check in with your energy, try following the 33-day method. If that only serves to make you feel trapped, guilty, or ashamed for not being able to stick with the plan, then please consider these 33 *ways* to tune into your energy instead of 33 days. **Structure can be so helpful until it isn't anymore. Use your best and kindest truth to discern when and how this works best for you.**

Section One: Introduction

Before you go through all the exercises it is good to know a little bit about how and why they work. In this section you will learn a little about me, and the what, why and how of what energy medicine is, as well as a brief introduction to polarity therapy.

Section Two: Getting to know your elements and chakras

Here you will find a chapter devoted to each element. These begin with personal stories of real life and real healing. The stories are meant to introduce you to the elements in a more contextual way. Each chapter contains information on its correlating chakra, altar suggestions, ways to bring each element into balance, and how to recognize when it's out of balance.

Section Three: 33-day Soul-Care Journey

This section consists of prompts, rituals, journal inquiries, and affirmations all laid out in five weeks of elemental cycles. This structure comes directly out of my online 33-day Soul-Care Challenge. There are no prompts on weekends other than the invitation to reflect and catch up, but If this linear structure doesn't support you then think of it as *ways* to balance your chakras and elements instead.

Section Four: Quick Reference Guide.

Easily and quickly look up the various imbalances associated with each chakra and the exercises that support each one.

There are three ways and infinite possibilities for how to go through this workbook.

1. The 33-Day Soul-Care Challenge

If you thrive on following a structure or are looking to cultivate more of it, you could go through the 33-day Soul-Care Challenge on your own or with the accompanying online course. There is an instructional video with each day's prompt and an entire community to go through the course with you. Learn more about joining the online course at: Elevationhive.com/soul-care-book

2. The quick reference guide

Check out Section Four at the end of this book for the quick reference guide. There is a list of common imbalances for each chakra where you can check your symptoms and choose the exercises within that elemental category that feel most resonant. Feel free to bounce around the book applying the elemental suggestions that meet your particular needs. Whether this is your first or fifteenth time going through the prompts, you can use this quick reference guide for continued support whenever you are curious about how your symptoms correlate to your energy system.

3. Think of this as 33 *ways* instead of days

Go at your own pace. Devote one week per element to go deeper. Read it backward. Take creative liberties and write wherever you want in the workbook, color outside of every line and find what resonates. Take the scenic route. Make up your own routine. **There is no wrong way to do it if it feels right for you.**

If you find that you are stuck, then reach out! I offer online classes, and even have a monthly membership (Hive) where you can find the support of like minds and grow exponentially on your path.

CHAPTER TWO: ENERGY MEDICINE

What is Polarity Therapy?

"The infinite within is ever becoming." - Dr Randolph Stone

Polarity is one of the most comprehensive and holistic systems of healing today. Rooted in the principles of energy medicine, Polarity is uniquely integrative in that it is energy work in the most ancient sense of "laying on of hands." Yet, it is so much more due to the broad scope of its founder, Dr. Stone.

Dr. Randolph Stone (1890-1981), was an osteopath, chiropractor, naturopath and mystic. His research, travel, and study of both Eastern and Western philosophies and modalities included Hermetics, Ayurveda, Chinese Medicine, Homeopathy, Naturopathy and European nature cures. Dr. Stone was a pioneer who created maps of the evolution of the soul through the body. He worked with the sickest and most "hopeless cases" with great results when everyone else had given up. Dr. Randolph Stones' extensive practice led to the creation of Polarity Therapy, a holistic approach to hands on healing. He called this approach Energy Medicine.

Through a variety of methods and applications, Polarity seeks to return the human energy field to a state of homeostasis. This could include but is not limited to yoga-inspired energy exercises, energetic nutrition, bodywork, craniosacral unwinding, reflexology and energetic communication/counseling. Polarity is transpersonal and evolutionary in its approach. It not only considers the micro perspective of the body and its functions, the psyche, and the emotions, but it is equally as interested in the macro view of the soul and the learning and growing we are here to experience. By focusing on wellness as opposed to just illness, we can put our attention on the whole person, finding out where their greatest resource lies. Rather than merely asking, "what is wrong with you," we can inquire as to, "what is right with you." Then we can work to align the system with the resonance of health that already exists.

Healing is not always the same as fixing. There are no accidents, as everything we attract, whether we see it as good or bad, could be viewed as an opportunity for personal growth when we honor the inherent intelligence of each individual and their unique healing path.

Energy medicine treats dis-ease at the vibrational level from where the dysfunction arises. In contrast, the Western allopathic approach tends to treat symptoms once they have already manifested. This view of illness as the enemy, seeks to combat everything on a strictly physical quantifiable level. Whereas the energy medicine perspective takes into consideration the experiential, psycho-emotional, karmic and unknowable aspects of the journey as well. It is holistic and preventative, ancient and cutting edge. There are many different modalities within the broader context of energy medicine, but the principals in this book are mainly based in Polarity Therapy which is heavily influenced by Ayurveda.

What is Energy Medicine?

"Energy cannot be created or destroyed. It can only be changed from one form to another." - Albert Einstein

At the atomic level we are made of the dance between protons, neutrons and electrons like everything is. You could say that at our most fundamental level we are nothing but impulses, frequencies and vibrations. We are elemental beings, inexplicably interconnected to all things, consisting of ether, air, fire, water, and earth.

There is a measurable electromagnetic field around the earth and around our bodies. Like the earth we have a positive, negative and neutral pole. Polarity works with the electromagnetic patterns expressed in the mental, emotional, and physical planes to determine where energy flows and where it is not flowing.

Within the polarity model, life energy could also be defined as the animating force, cosmic spark or breath of life, also known as "prana" in Sanskrit. It is our spiritual essence. Energy precedes matter. It gives rise to our physical structure, as well as our emotional, mental, and subtle layers of being. Life energy has its own intelligence that both affects and is affected by the digestion and assimilation of all of our experiences, beliefs, and perceptions.

Most simplistically, you could say that when energy is blocked, illness or disease arises. When our energy flows freely, we experience health and vitality. This is true, but of course it is simultaneously true that health from a holistic perspective is a dynamic complex journey that is not so black and white.

When we endeavor to work with our symptoms or circumstances at the energetic level, we recognize that life itself is the medicine. This isn't always the thing that brings us the solution or cure. Rather, the medicine is in the process of observing, acknowledging, learning from and acclimating to our ever-changing energetic matrix.

As a caterpillar goes into its chrysalis, its body begins to disintegrate as it transforms. You could say life is like that chrysalis. We are in a state of constant fluctuation and often it is not so pretty. We are becoming something new even when it appears that life is breaking us down.

What are chakras and elements?

The word *chakra* comes from the Sanskrit word *cakra* which means "wheel." The chakra system is made up of whirling energetic vortices that reside within the subtle body. There are between 7 and 114 chakras that can be addressed in Ayurveda but there are five primary physical chakras each with an associated element. They are the throat chakra (ether), the heart chakra (air), solar-plexus chakra (fire), sacral chakra (water) and root chakra (earth).

Our chakras and elements are always moving in and out of balance- orienting and reorienting to the various ways we are affected by the world and our experiences. Our subtle energy body is not static or stagnant. It is continually fluctuating based on our emotions, mood, thoughts, and things going on around and within us. It is not as cut and dried to say that our chakras are better off when they are open or worse off when they are closed. They are ruled by a dynamic and multidimensional mechanism that has its own rhythm, cycles and higher intelligence.

How do we work with the elements in the context of soul-care?

In my personal practice, I am always making adjustments to my self-care routines to accommodate the elemental energies that are moving through me. The language of the elements is poetry. It is symbology. I perceive this through my imagination, felt senses, the fleeting emotional states that I might otherwise dismiss if I was not taking the time to notice.

The elements are archetypal energetic frequencies. You can get to know your own elements by building rapport in the same way you would with any friend or relative- through conversation and attention. Connecting with your own energy body can be as simple as tuning in to your physical body and starting there. It is helpful to tap into your imagination and willingness to trust. If you have a hard time trusting your intuition, I have a free online course available at elevationhive.com/soul-care-book that helps to build your trust muscle to help you access your intuition through tapping into your imagination. Your imagination is the vehicle for your intuition, which makes intuitive development a creative process.

Balancing your energy elementally can be fun, as well as healing. As we learn to listen to how the elements behave and interact with one another, we can tell more easily how our chakras are affecting our experience and how our experiences are being processed through our energy.

There are ten-million ways to engage your elements and more practices than I could fit in this book. These are not necessarily the best they are just the beginning. But all roads lead to the same destination and every diversion has a purpose. Be willing to see this as an adventure and you can't go wrong! I encourage you to notice when you read about each element and prompt, what comes up for you. What words, images, or inquiries feel comfortable, safe, or exciting? Which ones feel annoying or uncomfortable or challenging? Noticing how you react can give you a clue as to where you tend to reside elementally, and where you may need to bring some healing or rebalancing.

This is both a science and an art of exploration. Your relationship with the elements is greatly enhanced when you are willing to pay attention and listen to what they have to say, by honoring the littlest things, slowing down enough to become a keen observer of your own energy, emotions, mind, and patterns. This is why engaging in and creating a daily practice is so powerful!

What are the benefits of developing a personal practice of working with your elements?

Sadhana is a Sanskrit word with over 22 variations on its meaning across various spiritual paths. From "magical procedures to attain worldly benefits" to a "method, or practice adopted to accomplish a specific goal." In the context of this book, you may consider your *sadhana* as a personal practice applied for devotional purposes. The devotion here is to *you* and your soul-care journey.

Practice is an essential aspect of any spiritual path. No matter how "go with the flow" you are or strive to be, there are innumerable benefits to having a consistent way to check in with yourself on a regular basis. The potential returns from doing this are tremendous. When you know yourself, you can track what is working in your life and what is hindering your progress. You can better assess when you are out of balance, and more quickly return to center when you flail.

Life is messy on purpose. How else do we get to burn through our karma, rise to the occasion or earn our chops? We are not here to attain ease and bliss in order to avoid the struggle. No amount of soul-care will give you a "get out of jail free card," I am sorry to say. As long as you are on the path of self-realization or personal development, there will always be challenges to meet and obstacles to face. *Having a practice to support you along the way is the best method to learn, track, hone, recalibrate and recapitulate in order to absorb and process life's lessons and trials.*

We may be down with the concept that energy precedes matter and form but learning how to work with it is key. When we continually loop around the same old issues over and over, manifesting the same caliber of life challenge, dis-ease, or relationship struggles, at some point, we have to take responsibility for how we are participating in creating our experience. There is power in bringing our patterns to consciousness. Often that initiates the shift on its own. But to truly change how the world is responding to us, we have to change our inner reality. Learning how to work with your energy is the best way to make these fundamental, long-lasting shifts.

Working with your elements provides a construct through which you can view the world, your idiosyncrasies, strengths and struggles. It provides a language, and a means to communicate with your energy system. By learning how to observe yourself, you can rewire the broken connections, heal your past, create a new path and find empowerment in each present moment. By cultivating these tools, you will make shifts on the subtlest levels that ripple out infinitely both backward and forward in time. Taking responsibility for your energy brings healing to not only your present moment self and all your relations but your ancestors and future generations on a quantum level as well.

The 33-Day Soul-Care process is not necessarily the practice itself. You may not use these exercises daily in this way. It is meant to offer an introduction to your energy system through Polarity principals, exercises, and chakra balancing tools. Polarity is a broad, holistic healing modality, but its principles can easily be applied to self-healing. With a basic understanding of how your energy organizes, you can learn to gather the medicine of the moment and find the precise recipe for the healing you need.

Each exercise in this book is intended to offer insight into how your energy is flowing. By learning how to listen, you will create your own relationship with your energy system, and your practice will evolve out of this. It is less about "what" you are doing each day and more about "how" you are related to what you are doing. How are you relating to yourself and your life? How are you listening to your body and energy? How is this working for you?

This sounds great but how hard is it going to be?

Over the years I have endeavored to create a personal practice that contains equal parts discipline and responsiveness to the moment. This means showing up no matter what to tune in and listen to my greater self. What is it that I truly need? How can I best align myself in order to really know? Often my "small mind" will try to convince me that sleeping in is actually beneficial. Not getting on my yoga mat each morning would be much easier. Not meditating when my brain is spinning would be calmer. Not sitting in the uncomfortable feelings when they are choking my throat chakra almost certainly *seems* better.

These voices will never cease to try and curb me from my practice no matter how deviant or untrue I know they are. They will still try to convince me. With practice, they get quieter though. With practice, they become more obvious to discern from my authentic truth. With practice, I can learn to have compassion for the parts of me that want things to be easy or automatic and make choices based on my highest good instead.

As we wobble our way to the light, we must embrace our shadow parts, our shady parts, our wounded parts and our subversive inner rebels. They all belong to the same soul family that is you. Creating a devotional practice means honoring yourself in the highest way possible with:

Radical self-acceptance

Deep self-love

Endlessly curious exploration

Rapt attention and fascination

Fierce determination

Surrender to and acceptance of your divinity.

The world is your mirror, every challenge a holy teacher, every day a new opportunity to remember that you are *worthy*.

SECTION TWO: GETTING TO KNOW YOUR CHAKRAS & ELEMENTS

CHAPTER THREE: ETHER

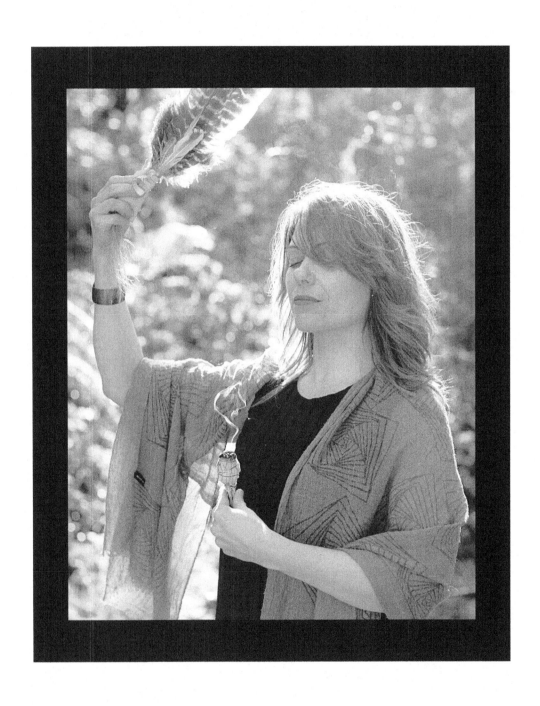

ETHER

Space

Sound

Form

Grief

The unborn

Star-filled nights and open vistas

Imperfections and reflections Choking notions

Om filled oceans of renewal space

Oneness and separation

The hollows

The bellows

The hallowed places

Whole

Spacious

Graciously

Returning

To center to

Now

Flying through Infinity

Sparkling with Purity

Vibing with the Frequency of

Luminosity

Invoking

Yoking

All things

No things

The creative spark

stark

And empty

Full of neutrality

Unlimited possibilities...

Space

Spirit Communications and Dream Initiations

Back in 2009, a Q'ero Shaman and his assistants came to my town from the high Andes of Peru to connect the energy lines of the North and South. They offered a weekend workshop to share certain teachings that would establish an energetic connection between our two hemispheres, by offering the participants here in the North a transmission and a practice of working with the seven *Nustas* or Goddesses of South America. I knew about the workshop because it was located at the wellness center where I had an office for my private healing practice. At the time, I did not have the money to go to the workshop, so I didn't think much about it.

My mind was soon changed, however, when I had a dream a few days before the workshop started that completely changed my life in a powerful way. In addition to affecting my decision about participating in the workshop, this dream was an initiation into a way of working with dreams from a waking state that I had not been engaged in prior. Shortly after this incident, however, I began studying and practicing dreamwork and this method of communicating with my dreams has since become a pillar in my work both personally and professionally.

In this dream, a group of unfamiliar Peruvian people came to my door. They were peeking in my windows and wandering around my yard. They seemed harmless but I was afraid to let them inside. They continued to knock on my door. I tried to hide inside my house and told them to go away. They yelled through the door that they knew I had some stones of theirs, but I didn't know what they were talking about or where the stones were. When I woke up, I was confused, but I knew the dream was important.

It was so vivid that I couldn't let it go. I asked for a friend's advice while we sat outside in my backyard. Calmly, they proceeded to dismantle my house piece by piece while I frantically looked around and tried to figure out if I had the stones they were talking about. I discovered to my surprise that the stones they were looking for were hidden underneath my mattress. When I woke up, I was confused, but I knew the dream was important. It was so vivid that I couldn't let it go. I asked for a friend's advice while we sat outside in my backyard in the sun, and she suggested I find someone who knew how to work with dreams to help me interpret what it meant. I decided to try on my own, so I went into a meditative state and re-entered the dream right then and there.

I closed my eyes and imagined myself back inside the dream standing in my home. I answered the door this time and asked the woman point-blank why she was there and why they were dismantling my house. She told me once more that I had the stones they needed, and I was supposed to go to the workshop that was happening that weekend. I told them I didn't have the money, and she said not to worry, the money would come.

Oddly enough, I got an unexpected check in the mail that week for almost the exact amount. Of course, I knew it was no coincidence. The next day, I went to the woman who was hosting and organizing the workshop and asked if it wasn't too late for me to come. She said I was welcome to join them, but there was one prerequisite that everyone was required to do beforehand. **I had to find seven stones and bring them with me!**

At the time, I did not know whether my participation in this workshop would mean anything or not. I didn't know if it would change me, or if it would empower me to help bring change forth in the world. But within the workshop there was a moment when the Q'ero Shaman asked each of the participants in the workshop to approach him in the center of the room, one by one. He held a feather in his hand and waved it around in front of our throat chakra where the ether element resides. I felt completely neutral at the moment when I got up to take my turn in the center of the circle. But as soon as he started waving that feather in my throat chakra I felt a tremendous surge of energy pour through me. I let out a blood curdling scream at the top of my lungs that I am sure must have startled the other 50 or so people in the room. I did not have any control or even self-consciousness. Afterwards, I felt incredibly empowered. Within a couple of years, something had indeed started to blossom, and miracle has followed miracle ever since.

One of the most important shifts that occurred for me as a result of this connection and opening of my throat chakra was the impetus to start paying more attention to my dreams. Once this doorway between the worlds opened up for me, my creativity burst forth, and I began painting visions that came in both waking and night dreams. I started writing from my dreams. I received songs, dances, and poetry from my dreams. These connections exploded all around and within me. I wanted to learn more about the creative unconscious, so I studied hypnotherapy, tarot, worked with an amazing, wonderful shamanic practitioner who became my mentor, and attended workshops with Robert Moss, including his Active Dream Teacher training. I started participating in the collective dreaming of the world in a more empowered way by offering sessions and classes both online and in person to support others tapping into their dreaming abilities.

Through paying attention to my night dreams, making space for conscious dream journey work and taking time out of my days to honor the visitations, inspirations, symbols, images, and emotions that come up, I have not only become an active participant in a running dialogue with spirit, but I have become engaged in the dreaming of my waking life in a more direct way. The most important thing I learned from doing this work for myself, with clients and students, is that we can all dream in magical, meaningful, powerful ways. Dreaming is not a rare skill reserved only for a special few. For as long as people have been on the planet, they have been dreaming. In many societies, throughout time and across the globe, communities have dreamed together. Dreams offer us wisdom and warnings. They inform us in a multitude of ways. All it requires is an open mind and a willingness to remember.

Of course, DreamWork is also a practice that is cultivated through regularly engaging, paying attention and honoring what comes. Because dreams are multi-dimensional, we need to approach them in creative ways. We must be willing to listen with more than our minds. We must learn to listen with our bodies, hear with our souls.

Trying to make dreams fit into our logical realm is like trying to stuff the universe into a small box that we can label and set on the shelf. Neat and tidy? Not so much. But it is possible to meet your dreams halfway between the conscious and subconscious realms. I cannot begin to tell you how many times I have had dreams that seemed odd, nonsensical, or meaningless and trivial, only to be utterly blown away by the powerful realizations and transformations they contain. I have harvested incredible wisdom and guidance this way. By cultivating curiosity and a willingness to pay attention, our dreams can inform us on so many levels.

DreamWork relates to the ether element (and in some ways the water element as well). Ether is the bridge between the conscious and unconscious realms. It is a way we can access our unlimited higher knowing and guidance through *direct communication with Spirit.*

Opening the gateway between this reality and what the shamans call non-ordinary reality, is how our higher spiritual centers can inform our lower ones. This kind of communication has informed my life in more positive tangible ways than anything else ever could. By learning how to listen and work with my dreams, I have found new outlets for creative expression and greater clarity around my purpose. Through DreamWork I have found tremendous healing physically, emotionally and spiritually. I believe that this is available to most anyone. If you have the interest and desire to explore them, your dreams can open up new worlds and unlimited possibilities for healing. They can also help to ignite and balance and empower both your ether element and all of your upper chakras.

About the Ether Element

Ether correlates to the throat chakra, which in Sanskrit is *Vishuddha*, meaning purification. The seed sound is "Ham." In Polarity Therapy, ether can be balanced physically through the joints and cavities of the body and the jaw (TMJ specifically). Science has proven, our physical bodies consist of 99.9% space. Our atoms are literally dancing around, creating the illusion of solidity. If you tap into this truth, you might notice your sense of self expanding. You are space, and spaciousness exists within and all around you. Your ether element is the gateway to Spirit and the upper chakras. It is the hoop of the medicine wheel. It is represented by the color blue and is accessed by looking out at expansive views. You can feel it in the cosmos as it sparkles into an infinite star scape, or from a vast cloudless blue sky, or the vantage point from a mountain top where everything is visible for as far as the eye can see.

In Polarity Therapy, all things have a positive, negative, and neutral pole, including each of our elements and chakras. The negative pole relates to our yin aspect and the positive pole to our yang aspect. There is nothing inherently wrong with the negative pole. However, it can be referred to this way interchangeably. From here forward, the positive pole in this section of the book will refer to "balanced" and the negative pole will refer to "imbalanced."

The positive pole of ether

When in balance, the ether element is fully expressed. It is comfortable in silence and feels spacious, sacred, empty yet whole. We can access profound bliss from this place. When everything is open and oriented to center, there are no blocks or illusions of separation to the infinite, fully present. Ether is patient, wise, humble, unattached, neutral. Ether knows total Equanimity. It knows it is connected to all things: Spirit, source, freedom, peace.

The negative pole of ether

The ether element can go out of balance in either excess or deficiency. When one has too much ether, the quality of spaciousness can be disorienting. There can be a disconnect from the body. Spaciness. This could manifest as an obsession with the non-physical world, dissociation, or soul loss. There could be a separation from reality, lack of boundaries, an inability to hold on to things or find stability. An ether imbalance could feel like too much freedom, wandering, separation, isolation, or losing the ability to be functional or participate in a balanced way within society.

When there is a constriction in the throat chakra or an ether deficiency, one might feel grief-stricken, lonely, confined or bound. This could manifest in the body as inflammation, arthritis in the joints or blocked bodily cavities. There could be issues with teeth, TMJ, the thumbs or big toes. Not enough ether could manifest in losing one's voice or not feeling capable of speaking one's truth. It could show up as a fear of silence, of speaking, or on the opposite extreme as the inability to listen to others. It could mean one cannot easily communicate with others or trust in their own intuition. Often this could cause extreme tension, apathy, feelings of disconnection from Spirit or feeling trapped.

Working with your ether element: Inquiry

You could try fasting for a day or even for a meal. Notice the sensation of emptiness in your stomach. It can be good for the body (sometimes) to take a break from eating so that all your energy that is normally diverted to digestion can be used to repair and heal your other organs and systems. It is also an excellent experiment just to notice your relationship with emptiness.

Eat some blueberries. Eat something light and chew very slowly with intention. When you eat with intention and mindfulness, tuning in to how it feels in your mouth and body, food can be healing not only for your body but also for your energy body.

Because ether is the first and highest vibrational chakra in the physical realm, it is considered the place of invocation. When we invoke something, we are tuning in to a higher source or consciousness and opening a doorway between this world and the world of Spirit.

As a practice, it is very powerful to take a few moments first thing in the morning (or right before bed or whenever you can fit it in) to create some spaciousness, to sit in silence and to invoke this kind of attunement to your higher self, or to "the god of your heart."

For your altar

The ether element is considered in some ways to be the altar itself. If you wanted to place things on an altar to represent ether specifically- you could meditate on the negative spaces where there are no things present or place an empty container to represent this. Ether could be represented by stars, galaxies, spacious blue skies, clouds, feathers, anything blue, or anything that represents source or Spirit to you. The shape is a circle and the seed sound you could chant to balance ether is HAM.

Stones that work well for balancing ether

Lapis Lazuli, turquoise, sodalite, blue agate or kyanite.

Working with your ether element: Exercise

Contemplate your relationship to your ether element by closing your eyes and tuning in to your throat chakra. Notice how your body feels. Notice what images arise. Open your eyes and list the first five-ten words or statements that come to you:

Which of these words or statements feel good to you?

Which of these words, statements (or anything about ether), invoke feelings of fear, sadness, resistance or disdain?

Finish the following sentences

If I had more ether I would...

If I had less ether I would...

If my ether was balanced I would...

CHAPTER FOUR: AIR

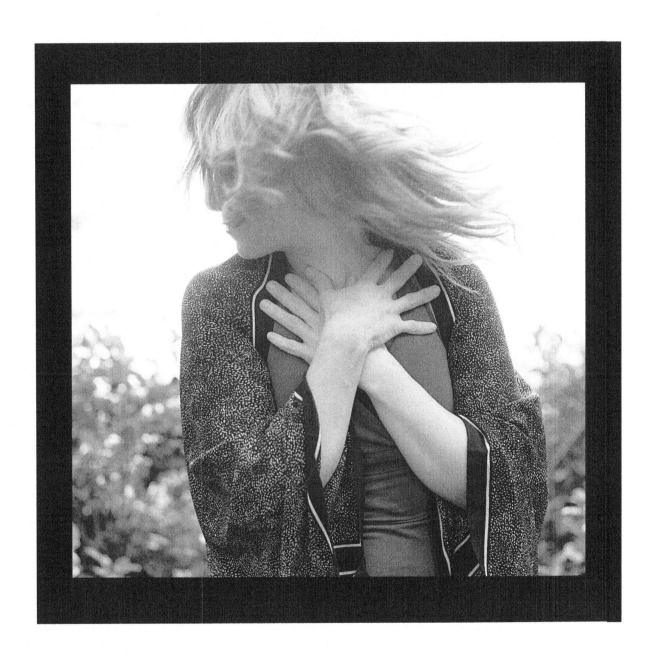

AIR

Unstruck

How we swoon and flatter Feathers flocking

(Alone/together)

Communal endeavors that heal and restore

Promises of forevermore

Spring is breathing hearts are beating Like a drum

Seeding our dreams of greener grasses

(I am/we are)

Starlight so

bright

Happily ever after

Mind over matter

New

Fresh

Restored

Rebirthed

From the heart of the earth

To the greatest heights

Flights of fancy Free

(you/me)

whirling through eternity

The Great Balancing Act

Years ago, when I was in the process of dissolving a significant relationship, I had a dream that seemed to sum up the journey of the heart to me. I saw two figures walking carefully across a tightrope high above a cavernous drop between two cliffs. They each held onto a long pole for balance. They were working together in a coordinated way, equally as in tune with each other's movements as they were with their own and the wind and the tightrope below them. This dream was showing me a metaphor for partnership. Love as the ultimate balancing act.

When we open ourselves to love, there is always a risk of falling. And it takes tremendous faith, cooperation, communication and courage to walk the tightrope of our heart with another. I love this metaphor for traversing the terrain of the heart chakra, as it pertains to so many aspects of the air element in general, even beyond romantic love.

There is a balancing act that happens whenever we open ourselves wide to any meaningful pursuit and attempt to cross the gap of inner growth. Often, we are then coordinating with different aspects of ourselves to get across. The internal communication between our body, mind, emotions, and environment requires another kind of balancing act altogether.

The French word for heart is *coeur*, which has its Latin roots in the word courage. There is no doubt that it takes tremendous courage to live from the heart. It is a vulnerable thing to be so high up in the air. To put ourselves "out there", for another person, for our passions, or for any endeavor that we care deeply about. When we are trying to convey our truth, we speak from the heart. Often this can cause palpitations, sweaty palms, anxiety, and nervous energy. In polarity therapy, all of these bodily functions are ruled by the air element.

About the Air Element

Air correlates to the heart chakra which in Sanskrit is *Anahata* which means unstruck. The seed sound is "Yam." The heart chakra is represented by the color green, and the six-pointed star, which is made of two triangles intersecting.

The heart chakra divides the upper energies from the lower- the spiritual from the physical. The upward triangle is the upward flow of energy evolving, and the downward-pointing triangle is the energy that is involuting or descending from the etheric plane into physical form as it moves from higher to lower vibrational states. This is the cycle of life. The heart chakra lies at the center of it, navigating the flow between the upper world and the lower; the etheric and the physical. It is the communication center between the two.

Our energetic system is constantly moderating and organizing itself around the input we receive across the multifaceted layers of our being. Life is a journey, and the best way to heal is to tune in to what your unique energetic balancing act requires of you in each moment.

As the wind changes, as the other characters around or within us shift, we have to make accommodations. To truly be in balance, we must constantly be willing to fluctuate, recalibrate, open, and close as needed. It is true for each of our energy centers that we will have times of bursting wide open and times of contraction. But the heart, in particular, is a tricky vortex of complex potency. This is why we grieve our losses and heartbreaks in cycles and layers. The heart moves in spirals, and growth is never a linear path.

Sometimes we need to clamp down in our heart center, to go through a dark night of the soul. This may be the only way to source the healing we ultimately need. We may need to fall into the cavern and let our heart shatter into a million pieces in order to hone our true resilience. It is only through our brokenness that we come to realize our wholeness is unconditional.

The positive pole of the air element

When in balance the heart is open and flowing, clear and focused. The heart rules the mind and its mental functions, patterns, loops and inspirations. Communication is flowing and automatic, writing, and conveying information happens efficiently.

The negative pole of the air element

Sometimes you can tell if you have too much air, or that your air is out of balance in an excessive way, when your mind is spinning. Maybe you feel a little "air heady", or perhaps you even have physical congestion that manifests in headaches or dizziness. Often someone with excess air communicates in a high-pitched fast-moving tone. Or their thoughts move so fast they jump from topic to topic without stopping to catch their breath.

When there is a deficiency, it is often experienced as contraction. Your heart chakra could feel tight or heavy. This might manifest physically as chest pain, difficulty breathing, upper back pain, shoulder pain, kidney or adrenal issues. Emotionally this might bring up issues of envy, jealousy, fears of inadequacy or feelings of not being enough. This can manifest as stinginess, backstabbing, gossip, a lack of integrity, or poor communication.

When your air element is "out of balance," it can be helpful to meet yourself where you are. What if being out of balance is ultimately just the recalibration you need to find your way? Rather than asking the tornado to stop spinning or expecting a fresh breeze to come out of nowhere into a stuffy locked up room, it is helpful first just to acknowledge that something is off. Hold space for what is uncomfortable or painful or just not working well.

When we approach our healing from a place of trust in the inherent intelligence of our dynamic soul path, we create more possibilities. More room for accepting that life is just a process of moving through layers and obstacles and lessons that we are meant to experience. So often, this can be enough to help the excess energies begin to dissipate on their own, or the lack of flow begins to breathe itself into better alignment again.

Working with your air element: Inquiry

Levity is great medicine. The air element loves free movement, play, and laughter. Spinning in circles, watching a comedy, or doing some laughter yoga can all help balance and uplift your air element.

Air is light and quick

Since air doesn't much like to sit still, it can be a fun exercise to allow yourself a moving meditation to tune into its light and agile qualities. Try spinning in circles or run in place for a minute and see how it feels to get things moving. Spend some time watching your thoughts to discover how your air is manifesting.

Is your mind quickly changing, distractible, or hurried? Do you tend to talk fast or use a lot of words? Do you express yourself with your hands? If so, it can be helpful to gently observe whether you feel you could use a little more or a little less air.

If you feel an aversion to quickness, high-pitched voices, or experience a lack of tolerance for others who display qualities associated with the air element, this may indicate that you have an air imbalance yourself. If so, it can be helpful to gently observe whether you feel you could use a little more or a little less air.

Air love's touch

Air is associated with the nervous system and responds well to touch. Sometimes just combing your hair or receiving a gentle shoulder rub can be very beneficial for the air element. In the Polarity therapy model, air manifests in the shoulders and chest or upper back areas, kidneys/adrenals, ankles, and is also connected to the skin. Forgiveness is a powerful heart chakra balancing tool.

Think about someone you envy and forgive yourself for your hard feelings. Think of someone who you feel has done you wrong and write a forgiveness letter. You do not have to mail it. You could speak your heavy-hearted unspeakable truths out loud and ask the air element to carry them away for you. Take some deep breaths. Repeat. Repeat. Repeat.

For your altar

Air is best represented by wind chimes or things in the air itself. You could use anything green or pink, heart-shaped or starshaped. Feathers, roses, or other flowers, or anything that represents love to you. Air loves humor and lightness, so bubbles or toys that fly through the air, a paper airplane, bird, angel or any flying object will suffice.

Stones that work well for balancing air

Green aventurine, emerald, rose quartz, prehnite, peridot or jade.

Working with your air element: Exercise

Contemplate your relationship to your air element by closing your eyes and tuning in to your heart chakra. Notice how your body feels. Notice what images arise. Open your eyes and list the first five-ten words or statements that come to you:

Which of these words or statements feel good to you?

Which of these words, statements (or anything about air), invoke feelings of fear, sadness, resistance or disdain?

Finish the following sentences

If I had more air I would...

If I had less air I would...

If my air was balanced I would...

CHAPTER FIVE: FIRE

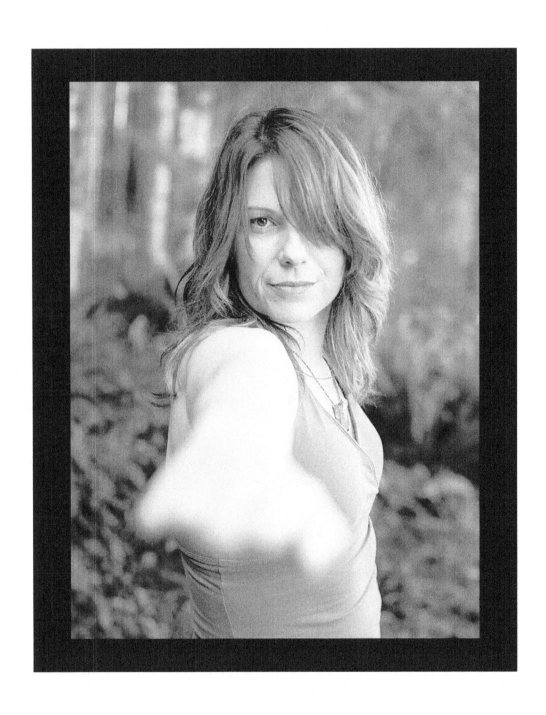

FIRE

I am

furious action

never tempted by distraction. My will

My bow & arrow

My quill

I am

the visionary

Master of my destiny

Sharp loud fast strong

I long for new beginnings Spontaneity

To live wild and free chaotically

Crazed and delicious

I am

Burning through the yearning

Flames devouring

Destroying

Giving, taking

With sparks that fly

I am

The war cry

The eye of the storm

The gaze warm

And bright as the sun

my power propelling my light

Compelling and free

I Devour and

Delight as you Cower before me

I am

the bow

the arrow

righteous action

Never tempted by distraction or desire

I am

fire

Fire of the Earth and Sun

We are made of each of the elements, but we all have a main constitutional element that tends to rule the show. For me, it is fire. And I can't think of an element I love more.

I loooooove tapping into my fire because it is the most courageous and creative resource for me. It is spontaneous and powerful. Dynamic and destructive. It gives, and it takes. It makes and destroys. It doesn't apologize for anything. Ever.

I have studied fire and cultivated my relationship with it elementally through meditation and observation, by lighting a candle on my altar or creating ceremony outside alone or in sacred company. Perhaps it is my favorite elemental ally because of how it helps to balance out my watery Cancer nature. Or maybe it is my Leo rising that draws me in.

I love the rush that comes from tapping into my ambition and diving into a new creative project. I love how fire empowers me to wake up early, take inspired action, and to get things done at the last minute with gusto, vibrato and a little bit of healthy anxiety.

One thing I have learned in the process of observing and working with my own fire is that there are many versions of it that exist, however, and not all of them are healthy. For instance, there are hearth fires that give us warmth and nourishment, and then there are forest fires that devastate homes and habitats. These various types of fire exist outside as well as inside us metaphorically, energetically.

Being out of balance could mean a lot of things. For me, it means that my fire tends to burn too hot, too quick. I have this habit of starting things, but in the past, I rarely had the gumption to finish them. No matter what. And this drove me crazy! So I worked with my fire to find out what other elemental qualities would help to harmonize and balance these tendencies.

As I took the time to tune in, I learned that it was a sustained fire that I was seeking. I wanted a fire that would burn in a contained and steady way, without taking over or fizzling out. I meditated on these qualities. This led me to connect with the fire that resides in the core of the earth. I realized it was a dependable, cultivated, predictable fire that I was seeking.

The fire of the earth is steady, impeccable, indistinguishable, and yet safely contained. After some time of cultivating my earthy fire, however, I realized I needed another element to give it more power and visibility. So, I tapped into my solar energy. I brought in the fire of the sun for its magnetic, bright, enduring, life-giving nature.

Together this combination has felt so deeply satisfying. Alchemizing. By working with these energies, I have found my fire balancing itself more readily. I have to tend to it continuously and remain consciously related to it, as I change. But this is the work of being a tender of one's energy. It is creative, ever-evolving, revealing and oh-so empowering.

About the Fire Element

Fire is the element of the solar plexus chakra, *Manipura,* which means 'lustrous gem' in Sanskrit. The seed sound or chant is "Ram." Fire is all about will and ego, power, our physical embodiment, and the way we take action in the world. It is represented by the colors yellow or gold like the sun. Fire expresses itself physically through our eyes and forehead, where we envision and focus on what we want to call in. It rules our fiery digestive functions, the alchemical powers within our bodies to break down food and turn it into fuel. It governs the strongest muscles in our body, the thighs that animate our ability to take action or run.

The positive pole of fire

Fire is the strength that propels us. That ignites our quick-twitch muscles that carry us the distance. Fire helps us orient to our future, to what we want to create and how. When we connect with our fire, we get clear on what we need to do and what action we want to take. Fire then fuels us to make it happen. Whatever we take in from life, whatever we receive, fire consumes it, transmutes it. Fire gives us the energy and power we need to wield our magic wand and manifest strategically.

The negative pole of fire

When we have too much fire, we tend to be inflammatory. Either physically, mentally or emotionally. We could become bossy, power-hungry, controlling, or overly focused on doing, on being seen or acknowledged for our successes. It can feel like ego. It can come out in violent outbursts.

Fire is also feared. We are usually not taught how to work with it; how to channel our anger or rage safely and effectively. So often, it eats away at us from the inside. If we do not honor or express ourselves or our power, then it becomes destructive externally or internally. These imbalances energetically could manifest physically as rashes or heartburn, eye or thigh problems. Sometimes we find that we can't stop running from here to there, or we can't start or finish anything effectively.

When we are deficient in our fire element, we might tend to give our power away. Sometimes when we lose essential parts of ourselves to life, to other people, to our traumas, then we lose access to our will. This makes it more difficult to access the discipline of discernment we need to feel empowered. Fire deficiencies can limit our ability to be fully embodied, present or courageous enough to make empowered decisions or take the right kind of action.

Building a fire can be tricky if the conditions are too moist or windy. If we look at fire symbolically, when we are stuck in our emotions (too watery) or spend all our energy fixating mentally (too airy), then it is much harder to ignite into action. But once we step on the path, and our fire is lit, it is much easier to take the next step. Once the flames are finally alive and licking, it is just a matter of fanning the flames and feeding our fire strategically to keep it going.

Working with your fire element: Inquiry

Fire is related to your physicality. How strong, muscular, and agile are you? Do you want to bring more of this in? Should you enroll today in a couch to 5k challenge to get you going? Or take a break from the gym to tone down those giant biceps, so your t-shirt sleeves can fit better?

Fire and your activity level

Perhaps you have too much fire and need to slow things down a bit. If you are go, go, go, then contemplate how you could honor your fiery nature in a contained and gentle way. Think of sitting in front of a warm cozy fireplace instead of burning the village down. Or maybe you need to stoke your fire and get more active in general. Start the project you've been procrastinating on. Enroll in that class. Step into your power and BEGIN. Fire builds its momentum through the doing of things.

How do we give space for the expression of our inner explosions? Do we let the sparks fly when they need to healthily, or do we keep it bottled up and pop our cork inappropriately spilling like a fiery geyser or volcano?

Anger is natural, and in some cases, very appropriate. It needs to have a healthy expression. It also has the potential to be dangerous if we don't express it in an intelligent way.

Fire and personal power

Tuning into your fire, how does it feel to contemplate your relationship to your personal power, your physical activity level, your vision, and the ability to take action in your life? How is your anger these days? How confident are you? Where do you have trouble, or how are you brilliant at getting things started or envisioning your direction in life?

You could contemplate these things mentally, but that would be a bit on the airy side. In order to cultivate your fire, it is good to DO SOMETHING about your findings. If you notice that you've been sedentary and avoiding going on that walk- stop thinking about it and get up and walk out the door. This is fire. Take the action. Honor your fire by putting on some loud music and dancing ferociously. Let yourself get loud. Go a little crazy. Scream at the top of your lungs. Bang on a drum. Have at it in a safe and sacred way.

For your altar

The easiest way to call in fire is to light a candle. A yellow candle works even better. You could place something yellow on your altar or use an image or something with the design of a sun or flames. If fire feels red, orange, sassy or flashy to you then do not

hesitate to use your creativity here. Fire loves anything passionate, spontaneous and ingenuitive.

Stones that work well for balancing fire

Citrine, amber, yellow sapphire, pyrite or tiger's eye.

Working with your fire element: Exercise

Contemplate your relationship to your fire element by closing your eyes and tuning in to your solar plexus chakra. Notice how your body feels. Notice what images arise. Open your eyes and list the first five-ten words or statements that come to you:

Which of these words or statements feel good to you?

Which of these words, statements (or anything about fire), invoke feelings of fear, sadness, resistance or disdain?

Finish the following sentences

If I had more fire I would...

If I had less fire I would...

If my fire was balanced I would…

CHAPTER SIX: WATER

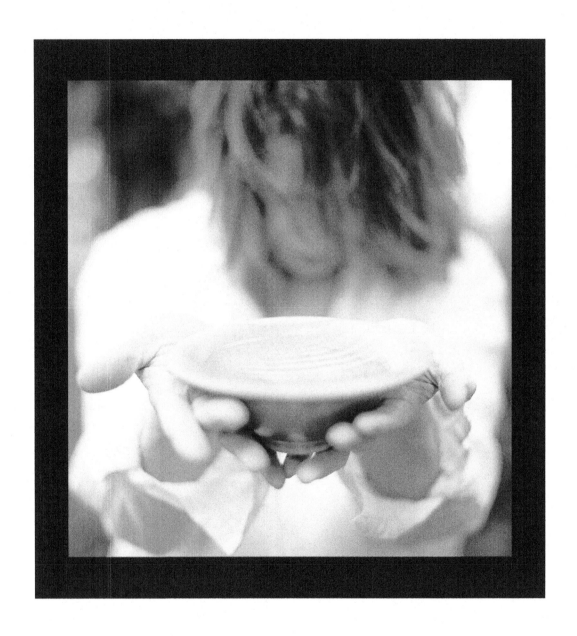

WATER

I sink down into the depths of my own pelvic bowl

Darkness envelops

the tears begin to flow Ah, water.

To be held and emptied

By the caress and storm of you

To be made old and new

Nursed and nurtured by the

Unknowable, unfathomable

Depths of you

until

Sweetly you release me

Into the silence of my belly

womb

Pleasantly savory, satiating,

Pulsating and pushing me

Into view of you

Sweet water.

Oceanic and rhythmic

Gushing, lapping, filling, emptying,

I am the flow that beckons to be let go

To know

Your depths and crevasses

You take me there

Into the mystery

Where I become the sea

Eternally bathed in unity

Until

(once again)

What was one

Becomes two

All

Because of you

Painting with Tears

A couple of years ago, I became aware that my fire element was causing me to work too hard, and my water element was being severely neglected. I was having a particularly difficult time letting go of my attachment to being productive. I wasn't allowing myself the space to chill out, have fun or play. All of these were gentle warning signs of an imbalance energetically.

To address this, I decided to hole up in my art studio with my best friend for three days and do an art project. I called it "a study of my water element." In fine art, a "study" means to sketch or make a rough rendering of a subject before you attempt to paint it "for real." As opposed to studying a still-life or anything external, I used my water element as the subject of my art.

I use DreamWork to source the imagery for all my paintings. When applied to this "study", the images I gathered for these pieces came to me from journeying to my second chakra in a meditative state also called Active or Conscious Dreaming.

I had several night dreams around that time as well, that revealed an old trauma and deep-seated grief residing in my second chakra that I had not processed because they had been lying dormant within my body and psyche. Bringing these things to my conscious awareness gave me the opportunity to process this energy through my art in a way that was potent, fun, and playful as opposed to only being painful.

I made three paintings that weekend. One of these paintings involved a woman's torso with bright orange Koi fish spilling out of it. I cannot tell you what that painting means to me on a conscious level, because I honestly do not know. I saw the image in my meditation, so I painted it. But as I began to paint it, I suddenly felt a surge of emotion welling up from "nowhere." I began to cry so hard that my tears spilled onto my painting.

I put more orange acrylic paint on the surface and used my tears instead of water to mix in the paint. I never needed any other water because I cried so much over that painting! I did not feel overwhelmed with sadness. I was not connected to the story around why the tears were there. But afterward, I felt so purged, light and hopeful. Using the water from my own tears as part of the medium I painted with was incredibly liberating.

I have since taught classes on painting this way, not necessarily from tears, but from the subconscious intelligence of our energy system. Our chakras communicate through symbols, images, emotions and sensations that can be accessed through our dreams, imagination, and creative unconscious. It is a powerful way to engage artistically.

I have made many paintings for my water element. I keep making them because I keep needing to do more work there. I stare at these paintings to invoke the feelings of flow and balance that I want to nurture in myself. I also visit water on a regular basis because I find it calming and centering. It cools my fire, moistens my dry earth, and quenches my soul every time.

About the water element

Water is associated with the sacral chakra, *Svadhisthana* which means 'one's own abode' or to take in pleasure, in Sanskrit. The seed sound or chant is "Vam". In polarity therapy, water imbalances can be reflected in the breasts or chest region, sex organs, bladder and feet. Also, we look at all the liquid systems in the body, such as the lymphatic system, tears, sweat or saliva. Water is all about flow, attachment, creativity, relationships, sensuality. It governs our inner rhythms and receptivity.

The positive pole of water

When in balance, our watery nature puts us in touch with ourselves, our bodies, and our generative ability to birth ideas, projects or even people. We are able to let things come and go easily. We can share what we have and receive what we need. We are able to harmonize with our deepest mysteries and our kinesthetic, intuitive gifts. We know how to play and express ourselves creatively.

The negative pole of water

In polarity therapy, water imbalances can be reflected in the breasts or chest region, sex organs, bladder and feet. Also, we look at all the liquid systems in the body, such as the lymphatic system, tears, sweat, or saliva.

When our water is out of balance in an excessive way, we find it hard to hold firm boundaries and might lose ourselves in other people's emotions. We could be overly empathic, finding it hard to differentiate what energetically belongs to whom. Or we may feel excessively emotional in general. Addictions, co-dependent behaviors, and overindulgence, in general, have to do with too much water. When our water is lacking flow, we can become fixed, rigid, too serious, or inflexible. We might be "all work and no play," or out of touch with our sexuality, creativity, or relationships.

Visiting water or even just consciously connecting with water can be balancing whether it is excessive or deficient. It can be helpful to use water to cleanse our energy. Swimming in saltwater works best, but sea salt or Epsom salts in a shower or bath works too.

Working with your water element: Inquiry

Your second chakra rules your ability to navigate relationships with healthy boundaries. Is there someone who asks too much of you? Or a way that you over give or feel undernourished? How are you relating to the people you interact with; the clients you serve, your colleagues, friends, loved ones, or partner? Notice how receptive you are to feedback or assistance.

How receptive are you in general? How creative are you allowing yourself to be?

How able are you to drop into childlike play with wild abandon?

How easy is it for you in your life or livelihood to give and take and go with the flow?

How able are you to receive pleasure or enjoy the sweet things in life?

Water goes with the flow.

Water teaches us how to move through even the tightest of spaces. How to ebb, and to flow, how to inhabit with grace the space we take up. When we allow ourselves to weep, sob, laugh until we cry (or until we pee our pants), we are engaging in our water element. When we choose to listen to our sensual nature, that too is engaging with water. Because water is related to our sexuality and our generative organs, this also contains the creative energy that brings anything to life. Drawing, painting, singing, dancing, or cooking are all ways to nourish your water.

For your altar

Although water is represented by the color orange, you could look for images of water or anything that relates to the various types of water that exist or feel nourishing to you. A fountain, a waterfall, a bowl of water, a shell, sea salt, seaweed or anything from the sea at all. Other altar items could have to do with relationships, giving and receiving, or receptivity. Water is associated with the hips and flowy movements, so a hula hoop or anything Hawaiian or tropical could also be used to represent the water element.

Stones that work well for balancing water:

Coral, citrine, carnelian, amber or orange moonstone.

Working with your water element: Exercise

Contemplate your relationship to your water element by closing your eyes and tuning in to your sacral chakra. Notice how your body feels. Notice what images arise. Open your eyes and list the first five-ten words or statements that come to you:

Which of these words or statements feel good to you?

Which of these words, statements (or anything about water), invoke feelings of fear, sadness, resistance or disdain?

Finish the following sentences:

If I had more water I would...

If I had less water I would...

If my water was balanced I would...

CHAPTER SEVEN: EARTH

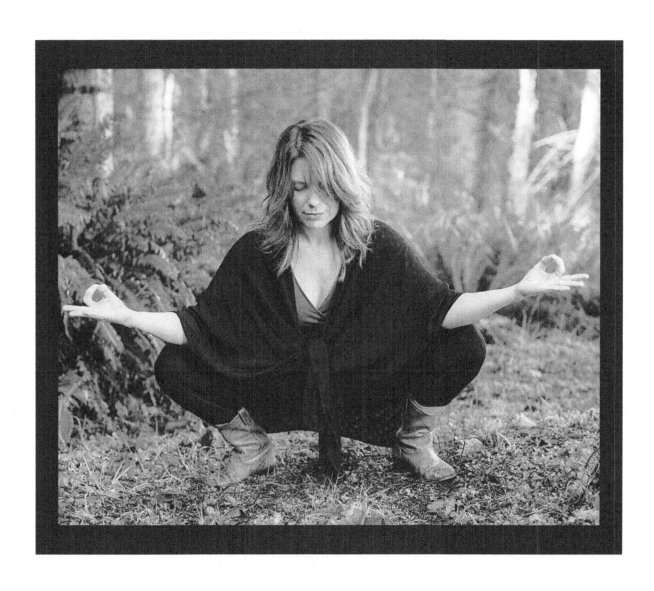

Earth

I am home

In the dark sweet cracks where the insects crawl over me

I am home

In dusty dawns

Where the wind remembers me

I am home

As I plunge my hands into the clay of your body

As I dance upon your belly

I am home

Under your stars

I gaze lovingly, adoringly

into your sky eyes

I am home

In the stillness

of stones who witness silently

I bow down reverently

So you will consume what remains of me.

I come from your molten womb

I return to your roots my tomb

May I be reborn

Through you

Infinitely

67

Growing Roots

When I was growing up, I often wondered what it would feel like to know in my body that I belonged somewhere. Due to this longing, I moved all over the country every couple of years throughout my twenties in search of a physical place that would give me the distinct feeling of being home.

During this gypsy roaming phase of my life, close to 20 years ago now, I moved to L.A, where I started my training in massage and polarity therapy at the Institute of Psycho Structural Balancing. At that time, I had recently become a single parent with two kids in preschool. I worked multiple jobs while going to school full time it was a particularly stressful time of my life.

I was continually experimenting with raw foods, cleansing, and fasting. Although this was all in an attempt to be healthy and "in tune," it had a very un-grounding effect on my energy and body. While I felt amazing in some ways, I also had no idea I was suffering from anxiety as I couldn't see the forest for the trees. I was in survival mode and unable to acknowledge how unstable I felt.

At the time that this was all escalating I knew I needed insight around my life. I was inspired to get a massage from one of my teachers which was a big commitment for me financially at the time. Thankfully, I made the investment. I did not expect, however, to have such a life-altering and profoundly healing session as I did. The interesting thing about this massage was that she never even worked on the majority of my body. All she did was touch my feet. For an entire hour! I did not mind, however, or even question her process. Because as soon as she lay her hands on my feet, I began to weep uncontrollably on her table. She lovingly massaged my feet while she spoke a little bit about the importance of home and family, and of feeling safe and secure. I had no idea how much emotional pain I had stored in my feet until she started to work it out of my muscles. I felt like I was crying for lifetimes of feeling lost, unsupported, and disconnected.

The entire hour flew past like it was 15 minutes, and yet when I got up off the table, I was no longer standing on the same two feet I had walked in on. As soon as I left her office, things started to shift in my life dramatically. I committed to myself that I would find a way to plant my roots. Even if I couldn't be in the "right" place, I would have to make the next place I landed my long sought after home no matter what. I was determined. Within a matter of months, I had moved myself and my two small kids back home to the Pacific Northwest into my very own home, where I started my practice in massage and polarity therapy.

I had always dreamed of living in an earthen structure. Serendipitously the one builder who I was referred to, to help me turn a garage in my home into my new office, just so happened to specialize in building cob and earthen structures. When I started my practice, it was in an earthen room with walls made out of clay that came from my own backyard. I sculpted a tree with visible roots into the corner of the room. I named my business Earth In Heart because I was intentionally calling in the earth element to help me plant my roots and establish a business that would give me security, abundance, longevity and a sense of belonging, place and community.

For the majority of the past sixteen years, I have worked in this room. Even as I write this, I am sitting under the tree I sculpted out of clay and hope, with my bare hands. Since then I have touched thousands of feet in this room and felt how the earth is expressed differently in every pair.

I could never have imagined how that one massage would inform me on so many levels. It taught me how impactful and life-altering physical touch can be, in combination with feeling so deeply witnessed and seen. It taught me how to know the difference between standing firmly on the ground and drifting aimlessly. But most importantly, I learned how invaluable one's relationship to the earth could be.

It has not been easy planting myself despite my persistent feelings of being out of place here. I've had to continuously cultivate my sense of home by tending my roots and my relationship with the earth element all these years.

Because earth energy is slow and steady, this quality has seeped into me incrementally over time. Each day, I feel my roots burrowing a little deeper and my soul getting a little lighter. Each day, I feel more at home inside my own body and soul, in communion with this planet that holds me and provides for me so abundantly.

I have learned from the earth what it means to be impeccable. I have learned how to show up day after day, year after year, being of service to the growth and healing of my clients, my children, and, most importantly, myself. The earth has taught me how to be in resonance with the deepest, most deliberate, and reliable resource I know. And how to find this within my body, in my own two feet wherever I go.

About the earth element

The Earth element is associated with your root chakra *Muladhara* which means "root" and "basis of existence" in Sanskrit. The seed sound or chant is "Lam." The earth element is all about beginnings, endings, planting, harvesting, crystallization, decomposition and letting things go. Birth, death, and all the cycles that take place in our bodies and in nature. Earth is the densest of all the elements as it is the last place energy arrives as it steps down from spirit to matter. In polarity therapy, we call this the involutionary journey. All things start out as energy, thought forms, vibrational essence. Eventually, if they are to become manifest, they make it to the earth plane. Here in the earth, things move much slower than they do in the air. If you throw a ball through the sky it travels pretty quickly. If you throw it into the dirt, not so much.

The positive pole of the earth element

When in balance, our earth element feels nourished and centered. We feel sturdy, grounded, capable, and stable. Earth rules our financial health, our ability to be supported, and taken care of abundantly. It allows us to feel a sense of belonging, connection, and resiliency.

The negative pole of the earth element

When our earth is out of balance it can become fixed and rigid, or very slow-moving. When we can't make a decision or make anything happen at all, sometimes it is because we are stuck in the earth.

Earth deals with our most primal instincts and often we hold fear around or change. Sometimes this manifests as low back pain or neck pain. Sometimes it means we are slow to do and would rather just be. If we are lacking some earth energy, we might have an aversion to its solid slow way. We might feel anxious, resistant, or irritatedd with its dense solid qualities.

Earth rules our digestive and eliminative functions. How well are you digesting your food? How is your relationship to letting things go either physically or emotionally? Sometimes IBS symptoms are rooted in earth imbalances and can be supported by energetically tuning in.

Working with your earth element: Inquiry

Go sit with a tree and imagine its roots. Or better yet, imagine your own roots growing out the bottoms of your feet or tailbone and connecting with the heart of the earth herself. How does it feel to connect with the earth like that? What do you notice?

If there is something you would like to let go of, you are invited to ask the earth to hold it for you or to transmute it into something new. The earth is happy to do it. It is just like composting!

How do you feel about balancing your checkbook? Taking the scenic route? Sitting still for long periods of time?

Eating dense or red foods, or things that grow underground like beets or ginger, are particularly nourishing for the earth element. The earth element is very important to attune to whenever you are embarking on a new journey or bringing something to completion. When we start off with both feet on the ground, in an organized, structured, and supported way, we are more likely to make it to our destination, by moving one foot after the other. With Steady intentionality. When we observe our relationship to the earth element, we invite a slowing down and arriving to happen. Orienting ourselves to the earth can feel stabilizing, centering, calming, and nourishing. It is our mother, it is our home, it is the place we come from and return to.

For your altar

The earth element is associated with the color red, with things made from our hands out of clay, things that are made from the earth, anything natural such as sticks and stones, or things that are dense or heavy. A potted plant or bowl of soil, some seeds, a drum, or a didgeridoo.

Stones that work well for balancing earth

Hematite, red jasper, smoky quartz, black tourmaline, bloodstone, onyx, garnet or ruby.

Working with your earth element: Exercise

Contemplate your relationship to your earth element by closing your eyes and tuning in to your root chakra. Notice how your body feels. Notice what images arise. Open your eyes and list the first five-ten words or statements that come to you:

Which of these words or statements feel good to you?

Which of these words, statements (or anything about earth), invoke feelings of fear, sadness, resistance or disdain?

Finish the following sentences:

If I had more earth I would...

If I had less earth I would...

If my earth was balanced I would...

SECTION THREE: 33-DAY JOURNEY THROUGH YOUR CHAKRAS & ELEMENTS

CHAPTER EIGHT: WEEK ONE

Welcome to the first day of the 33-day Soul-Care Journey. Whether you are here to engage in a sequential adventure over the next 33 days, or to explore on your own timeline how to balance your energy, it is good either way to begin at the beginning with ether.

Ether is the subtlest of the five elements as it is the gateway to Spirit and our higher energy centers. In the step-down process of energy coming into manifestation, or involuting as we say in Polarity Therapy, ether is the invocational element that we access when we begin any sacred process.

- If you desire to create a personal practice out of working with your energy by utilizing the "challenge" concept to support you in showing up for your intention, then the following suggestions may help you implement a structure. These are merely suggestions and are all entirely optional. Do what feels supportive to you!

- Set aside some time for yourself each day to do these exercises or to help establish a rhythm of engaging in some soul-care practices.

- Create a space in your home that you can come to each day where you can create a practice of tuning in. This could be setting up a new altar, reinvigorating an old one, or simply finding a place to sit each day as you tune into each element and record your experiences around working with your energy.

- Make a commitment to yourself to do this devotional practice. It takes will and discipline to maintain a practice.

- Get support or accountability by sharing your intention with a friend or family member, or within the accompanying online course.

- Be generous and gentle with yourself. If you fall off the wagon, stop the wagon so you can get back on. Be kind and easy on yourself to avoid self-sabotage.

- Keep track of your wins! Use the workbook, a journal or even a calendar to log what you do and what you notice. This is a great way to build awareness around what you learn and to acknowledge yourself no matter what.

Day One: Ether Element

Before we begin anything, whether it is a ritual, reading, session, project, etc. it is always good to have the utmost clarity around your intent and purpose. Today's prompt can be used to help you set the space for any endeavor you embark upon. As we are just beginning this journey together, your first soul-care prompt is to explore your "why" so you can get the most out of this book and these practices.

By focusing on how you want to feel and what you want to gain from an expanded perspective, beyond your ego's perceived limitations, you magnetize the highest possible outcome to you.

Find yourself a comfortable place to sit and tune in to your highest guidance for support. Allow yourself to do this exercise from a safe relaxed space and be willing to be curious about what comes. Do not force it. It can be helpful before you even begin reading the following section, to first close your eyes, take a few deep breaths and call in your personal guides, ancestors, allies, spirit helpers, God, Goddess, Spirit, Source, or whatever feels most aligned and supportive for you. You can also call in the five elements and four directions.

Ether = center

Air = East

Fire = South

Water = West

Earth = North

Today's Soul-Care Ritual/Prompt: Creating an Intention Statement

In the following exercise, you are invited to explore the reasons why you are here and what it would look like to create a personal practice of working with your energy. Why do you want to commit yourself to this 33-day challenge? Using free-writing, you will create an intention statement and affirmation that will help to guide and set the tone for your experience throughout.

Allow yourself to explore the following questions in writing. Freeform. First thought, best thought. Put your pen to paper or fingers to keyboard, and do not stop writing for a minimum of five minutes.

*What is your intention for beginning this 33-day Soul-Care Challenge?

*If you were to imagine the best possible outcome that could come from engaging in this work, what would that look like?

*What would it feel like?

Based on the free-write above, choose and circle six to eight of your favorite words.

From the words you gathered above, you will create an Intention Statement. An Intention Statement is like a mission statement and affirmation combined.

An Intention Statement starts with I AM and speaks in the present tense about the ways you want to feel and the things you want to become. It can be several sentences, but you want to make it concise enough to recall easily and recite regularly.

For example, I might write something like this in the first exercise:

My intention in taking this course is to learn how to balance my own chakras and tend to my energy, so I can take things less personally, have more energy and feel more powerful, centered and calm within myself and more patient with those around me. Ideally after going through this challenge if I could have anything I would know how to be more in tune with my energy, so I could be a better parent and healing arts practitioner. I would be able to tune into and trust my inner guidance more easily. I would have tools to make an effective, doable self-care practice, and I would continue to use them.

My favorite words from this are: Inner guidance, trust, patient, energy, powerful, practice, centered.

My Intention Statement: I am powerful, centered and patient. I know how to trust my inner guidance, and I have a personal practice that I engage in every day that helps me to stay centered. I am in tune with my energy!

*Write out your Intention Statement in the space below:

Now that you have created your intention statement, you are invited to place this on your altar, hang it somewhere visible, and speak it out loud daily if that feels supportive. You can always return to the exercise and redo it as often as you need in the future.

Daily Affirmation

Each day we will provide an elemental affirmation. Today you are creating it!

Daily Acknowledgment

This space is intended for you to write down something you accomplished that you are proud of. It could be that you completed the exercise, watched the video, wrote a reflection or honored yourself in another way. If you have not completed the activity for the day, simply write something loving or kind to yourself here and congratulate yourself for being alive!

Daily Reflection & Journal Inquiry

What did you notice when working with your ether element today? What felt nourishing to you? Did you have any resistance around it? use this space to reflect on your answers below.

Day Two: Air Element

The air element resides in the heart chakra and rules our ability to take in life through our breath. Our inhalation of air, breath and prana, all affects the nervous system and our mental-emotional faculties. Often when we feel anxious or mentally fixated, there is an air element imbalance at play.

Today's Soul-Care Ritual/Prompt: Breathwork

For today's Soul-Care prompt, you are invited to do some breathwork to open your lungs, chest, and tune in to how you bring air into and out of your body. The 4/7/8 breath is a great place to start. If you have other breathwork practices you prefer, or if you know *pranayama* (the yogic word for breathwork), you are welcome to try those as you mindfully connect to your heart chakra and air element. There are many physical, emotional and energetic benefits to doing breathwork. Some studies have shown that even starting with this simple framework, one can reduce anxiety and stress levels and improve sleep while decreasing fatigue, depression and even hypertension.

How to do the 4/7/8 Breath

Begin by letting all the air out of your lungs. Then <u>inhale</u> through your nose for **four** seconds, <u>hold</u> your breath for **seven** seconds, and <u>exhale</u> out your mouth for **eight** seconds. Do this several times. Notice how you feel! If it is hard to hold your breath for this long, you could do it for less time as long as you keep the same ratio such as 3, 3.5 and 4 seconds respectively. The more often you do it the more befits you will notice!

Suggested Daily Affirmation

I am grateful for my breath, and how it calms and centers me. With each inhale I take life in fully, and with each exhale, I let go of that which no longer serves me.

Daily Acknowledgment

What did you accomplish and/or how did you honor yourself today? What altar items did you choose? Document how you completed your daily soul-care ritual.

Daily Reflection & Journal Inquiry

What did you notice when working with your ether element today? What felt nourishing to you? Did you have any resistance around it? use this space to reflect on your answers below.

Day Three: Fire Element

The fire element resides in the solar plexus chakra and rules our will and our sense of personal power. This is also the place we go to energetically when we need to take action. When other people's energy intrudes on our own we can work with our fire element to clear and reclaim our personal power and sovereignty. When we feel resistance, anger, rage, or frustration we can work to clear that in our fire element as well.

Today's Soul-Care Ritual/Prompt: Cut Cords with the Woodchopper

For today's Soul-Care prompt you are invited to do a Polarity Therapy exercise to cut energetic cords, clear any negative emotions, balance your fire, and reclaim your energy. This energy exercise combines movement, sound and visualization. This Polarity Exercise is affectionately called the Woodchopper.

How to do the woodchopper exercise

Before you do this exercise, tune in to your solar plexus chakra and notice if there is something you want to release. Once you have identified what you want to let go of, imagine holding it in your hands. Using your abdominal muscles to protect your back and being mindful of your body, raise your hands overhead and bring them down as though you are chopping a piece of firewood. As you release your ax (or the emotion or energy that you want to let go of)-- contract your diaphragm making a loud "HA" sound.

Do this exercise three times loud and strong!

Suggested Daily Affirmation

I am courageous and powerful. I shine my light with confidence and clarity. My energy is clear, my body and being are sovereign, and I readily let go of any ties or unnecessary emotions or energies that do not serve me.

Daily Acknowledgment

What did you accomplish and/or how did you honor yourself today? What altar items did you choose? Document how you completed your daily soul-care ritual.

Daily Reflection & Journal Inquiry

What did you notice when working with your fire element today? Did you have any resistance around it? What felt nourishing to you?

Day Four: Water Element

The water element correlates to your second chakra also known as your sacral chakra. It includes your sex organs, lower abdomen, and low back. The water element affects your ability to be receptive, to be in relation to others, and it also houses your creativity and sensuality. Today's soul-care prompt is to be near water or visualize water and tune in to your own watery nature to help you balance your water element. Tuning into your water element can allow you to let go of attachments, go with the flow, and drop into your creative playful nature.

Today's Soul-Care Ritual/Prompt: Embody Your Water

Tune into your watery nature in an embodied way by finding some water to commune with!

How to connect with your water element

If you are able, we recommend visiting an actual body of water. The second chakra is very much about embodiment, so the prompt is to observe this body of water, watch how it moves and allow your body to move that way too. If you cannot go to a physical location with water, then consider taking a mindful bath or shower and connect to your watery nature as you bathe. Even drinking extra water and blessing it before it enters your body can become a healing ritual.

Contemplate how your thoughts and emotions affect water molecules, as Dr. Masaru Emoto discovered in his book The Hidden Messages in Water. Using this philosophy, treat the water inside of your body with intentional thoughts and words of adoration and sweetness as though you were speaking to a lover, friend, or pet. Be kind to your inner child today and revel in some kind of sensual joy, pleasure, and creativity.

Suggested Daily Affirmation

I let go of any unnecessary attachments with ease. I love my watery nature and nourish and treat myself with adoration and sweetness. I enjoy being in the flow of life.

Daily Acknowledgment

What did you accomplish and/or how did you honor yourself today? What altar items did you choose? Document how you completed your daily soul-care ritual.

Daily Reflection & Journal Inquiry

What did you notice when working with your water element today? Did you have any resistance around it? What felt nourishing to you

Day Five: Earth Element

The earth element correlates to your root chakra. This is your first chakra that relates to feelings of safety, predictability, financial and physical security, and physical wellbeing. In today's prompt, you will learn a polarity energy balancing technique to support you in tuning into your energy in an embodied way.

Today's Soul-Care Ritual/Prompt: Polarity Balancing

Today you are invited to tune in to the way energy flows through your body by balancing your positive and negative poles.

How to balance your poles: A Polarity Therapy balancing technique

To begin, you can either stand or lie on your side. You will place your right hand on the back of your neck at the base of your skull or occiput, and your left hand on your abdomen or low back, wherever is more comfortable for you. Pay attention to the sensation in your hands and the feelings that come up in your awareness as you do this. You are invited to bring your awareness to your body and notice any sensations, colors, images, or emotions.

The earth element is the densest and most embodied of all the elements. Notice how it feels to tune into your root chakra as you do this. Your nervous system should begin to reset and you will notice a calm grounded feeling coming over your body. You could try switching hands to see which direction feels better for you. The right hand is your positive pole which sends energy and the left is your negative pole which receives energy. Stay in this position as long as you would like.

.

Suggested Daily Affirmation

I am calm, centered, and balanced. I feel grounded, rooted and flexible like a tree. I feel safe, abundant, and sturdy.

Daily Acknowledgment

What did you accomplish and/or how did you honor yourself today? What altar items did you choose? Document how you completed your daily soul-care ritual.

Daily reflection & journal inquiry

What did you notice when working with your earth element today? Did you have any resistance around it? What felt nourishing to you?

Weekend Reflections

You are invited to go with the flow of your weekend and take time off from the challenge or use this time to catch up. To keep up your momentum, you may choose an element that needs more support or attention. Use the prompts below to tune into which element felt really good, and which one felt not so good.

Weekend Inquiry & Journal Prompts

What did you notice when working with all of your elements throughout the week? Did you feel or experience anything different or out of the ordinary, such as synchronicities or a new awareness?

Was there one element that you had resistance to more than the others? What about it was uncomfortable? Is there anything that you feel called to do to honor that or continue to work with it? What would it take for you to come into greater balance with this element energetically?

Was there one element that felt better than the others? What felt good about it? What happened or what did you notice in your body or life as a result of you tuning into this element?

How could you call on this element more to enhance your life and energy?

What is one thing you will do this weekend to honor your Soul-Care journey?

CHAPTER NINE: WEEK TWO

Day Eight: Ether Element

Ether is represented by space or the quality of spaciousness that exists within and around things. One way to work with the ether element is to bring things that are intangible into tangible form through images, symbols or objects. Creating a physical space for the sacred in your life and infusing this space with intention and love can be very nourishing for the ether element.

Today's Soul-Care Ritual/Prompt: Make a living altar

At the beginning of this soul-care journey, you were invited to set up a time and space for yourself to engage with your energy through the elements daily. Today's Soul-Care Prompt is to bring that into an even more tangible way by setting up a living elemental altar if you haven't already. If you do have an altar space, then today's prompt is to re-enliven your existing one by adding something new that acknowledges the elements so you can be interacting with them more intentionally.

How to set up a living elemental altar space

You can create an altar in any area you inhabit, no matter how small. It can include things that you already own, objects you find in nature or whatever feels sacred to you. It is nice to have a cozy corner or small cleared out area in your home that is private and clean to start. You could place a small table, nightstand, shelf or another surface down and use this as the focal point. An alternative if you do not have a small table or surface, would be to lay down a cloth, scarf, or even create a space outlined by stones. The main idea is to designate a place where you can put other sacred objects that have personal meaning to you.

In each of the elemental sections of this workbook, there are ideas listed as altar suggestions. You can use these as a general reference. What represents your version of the divine? What deities, ancestors, animal spirits or other higher beings help you feel connected, aligned or supported? Many items can help us tune into the sacred, such as crystals, stones, shells, fresh flowers, tarot or other oracle cards, a candle, a feather, essential oils, branches, leaves, moss or even a bowl of water. You could place a picture of each of the elements on your altar and rotate it daily, or just leave the ones you are most wanting to call in for greater balance.

What is a living altar?

I like to think of my altar as a living embodiment of the elements. The elements are sentient energies we can call upon, create relationships with, and get to know on a personal level. They have a soul, and your altar itself has a soul. You could imagine this as a dear friend who is here to support and hold space for you.

The more you interact with it, the deeper your relationship will be. Communing with your altar could mean touching each object, speaking to it, cleaning it, adding to it, or engaging in some way. This kind of attention, combined with devotion, is its own form of spiritual practice. There is no wrong way to do this. Feel free to make it up as you go!

Suggested Daily Affirmation

I am a divine being, connected to all life everywhere. My body is my temple, and the space I inhabit is a sacred sanctuary.

Daily Acknowledgment

What did you accomplish and/or how did you honor yourself today? What altar items did you choose? Document how you completed your daily soul-care ritual.

Daily Reflection & Journal Inquiry

What did you notice when working with your ether element today? What felt nourishing to you? Did you have any resistance around it?

Day Nine: Air Element

The air element resides in the area around your heart in the chest and shoulder region. When your chest is curved inward and your posture is lacking, it is harder for your energy to flow. By opening your upper back, chest muscles, neck muscles and spine, you create more space for the energy to circulate through your heart space. The functionality of your heart chakra is enhanced when you tap into feelings of love and gratitude. Putting these two things together can help to open, clear, balance and harmonize the energy in your heart chakra.

Today's Soul-Care prompt: Twofold Somatic Process

Today's prompt is a two-fold somatic process that is intended to balance your heart chakra/air element. The first part is through opening your physical body, and the second part involves visualizing and connecting with each of your body parts while invoking a feeling of gratitude and health.

How to do the twofold somatic process

The physical aspect of this exercise is intended to open your chest and spine. Doing this will also open the flow of energy through your heart chakra. The entire exercise will take about ten minutes to complete. It is not recommended to fall asleep in this position or to stay longer than 20 minutes. Modify as needed for you.

Begin by finding a bolster to place under your spine. The width of the material you use will determine how much physical opening you experience, so you are invited to start small and go bigger depending on what is right for you. You could use a rolled-up hand towel or bath towel, blanket, or foam roller and small pillow for your head, depending on how much opening is appropriate for your body. Lay on the ground or a yoga mat with the length of the bolster running vertically under your spine. Allow your arms to fall open naturally at your sides. Breathe, relax, and tune in.

You will now begin to tune into your body, visualizing and connecting to each of your body parts starting at your toes and working your way up. As you bring your awareness through your body, gently affirm out loud or in your head that each location is healthy and whole. Feel gratitude for how each body part and all your physical systems support you.

For example, you could say:

"Thank you, feet, for grounding me to the earth and helping me to move through my life."

"Thank you, knees, for helping me to take each powerful step on my path."

"Thank you, muscles, joints, blood and bones, for circulating, undulating and moving me efficiently and effectively through the world and all of my experiences."

Speak out loud if you can, honoring and thanking your body for functioning so well. If there is one part of your body that feels painful or does not function as well as you would like, you are invited to give it some extra love. Think of each of your body parts like they are your beloved children. Sometimes it is harder to love your problem child, especially when it is acting out or misbehaving, but they are often the ones that need it most. Be kind, loving, and affirming of your body's health and wellbeing as you focus on each individual area.

Daily Affirmation

I am so grateful for my physical body and the miracle of my being. I am healthy, whole, and vibrantly alive. I love myself exactly as I am.

Daily Acknowledgment

What did you accomplish and/or how did you honor yourself today? What altar items did you choose? Document how you completed your daily soul-care ritual.

Daily Reflection & Journal Inquiry

What did you notice when working with your air element today? Did you have any resistance around it? What felt nourishing to you?

Day Ten: Fire Element

Fire is active, creative, visual, embodied, and passionate. It rules the solar plexus chakra, which manifests physically in the center of your torso, eyes, and thighs. The fire element affects our ability to take clear and decisive action using our will and personal power. Often when we find ourselves wanting to do something, but we have resistance to getting it done, the fire element can be helpful to move that energy along.

Today's Soul-Care Ritual/Prompt: Conquer Your Resistance

For today's prompt, you are invited to take *action* around something you have resistance to doing. Easier said than done, I know! But bear with me, as I am going to share a short exercise that will help you with this.

How to tune in to your fire element and move through resistance

To begin with, you will place your hands on your solar plexus chakra and tune in. Imagine that it is open, balanced, healthy and strong. You can visualize a warm yellow-gold color emanating from this space. How does this feel? Is it too overpowering or barely limping along? Either way, just honor what you notice.

Know that by simply tuning into your fire element with clear intent, you can harness and access your will, discipline and personal power. It can balance itself just by receiving your focused attention and love. Everything you need is there. As you tune in to your fire you have the ability to access your will to become more decisive and empowered to take action. Visualize what this could look like. What would it feel like?

Now think of something that you want to do but have had resistance to or have been putting off. Then decide on one thing that you can do to move towards this. It could be starting a new project, picking up something that you have been ignoring, or it could be as simple as cleaning out a junk drawer or going and doing something physical like taking a walk or bike ride. By specifically doing something that you have been saying you will do but have been having a hard time actually getting to, you enhance your fire element and create more momentum for even the harder things to come forth with ease. Start with something small. Take only the first step at first.

Whatever you do, acknowledge and affirm that you are awesome and that whatever you did was enough!

Now your assignment is to go do it. Literally, get up and go now!

Seize the moment!

Daily Affirmation

I move through resistance with ease and potency. I am powerful and embodied. I take decisive action in the direction of my visions and goals.

Daily Acknowledgment

What did you accomplish and/or how did you honor yourself today? What altar items did you choose? Document how you completed your daily soul-care ritual.

Daily Reflection & Journal Inquiry

What did you notice when working with your fire element today? Did you have any resistance around it? What felt nourishing to you?

Day Eleven: Water Element

The water element correlates to your second chakra, which affects your sex organs, lower abdomen, low back, and feet. Water is the seat of your generative abilities, including your creativity. By tapping into your creative potential, you are able to enhance your second chakra.

Today's Soul-Care Ritual/Prompt: Allow Your Creativity to Flow

Today you are invited to honor your water element by engaging in and exercising your creative genius through a playful exploration so that you can allow your creativity to flow through you. But before we begin, you must first forget about any preconceived notions you may have around whether or not you are creative. Just suspend all judgments.

You can do this by tuning in to your second chakra. Coming into a relaxed position, bring your attention inward. Feel into your sacral or abdominal region where your second chakra resides. Imagine you have access to unlimited amounts of inspiration and creativity in this part of your energy body. No matter how creative or not creative you think you are. If you have a hard time accepting this as fact then I want you to remember one thing: **You were once a spirit being made of pure energy who magnificently manifested a physical body, which takes tremendous creative power.**

You started out like everyone else, as potential energy entering into form via your mother's second chakra! The water element that nourished you from inside the womb you came from was your very first home. You belong to the water. And even now it makes up over 50% of your physical being.

For the purposes of this exercise, you Since you incarnated, you have created all kinds of things. Your life is a creative project that is ever unfolding. It is your birthright to tap into this. For the purposes of this exercise, you are invited to take pleasure in exploring your creativity without any expectations. You do not need to make something beautiful or perfect. You only need to explore the feelings energetically that come up as you engage in your creativity. *This is about the process, not the product.*

How to balance your second chakra through tapping into your creative juices

As Julia Cameron shares in her book, *The Artist's Way:*

> *"Art is an act of tuning in and dropping down the well. It is just as though all the stories, painting, music, performances in the world live just under the surface of our normal consciousness. Like an underground river, they flow through us as a stream of ideas that we can tap down into. As artists we drop down the well into the stream. We hear what's down there and we act on it—-more like taking dictation than anything fancy having to do with art."*

There are unlimited possibilities for how you can tap into your creativity. Arranging a bouquet, writing a poem or story, drawing or doodling, coloring, or painting are all great ways to access the flow. When you do this with the intent to connect with your water element, energy will begin to move through your second chakra in a new way.

One of the most accessible creative outlets for the second chakra is cooking since making food is something you most likely need to do anyway. All you need for this to become a fun and even sensual way to express your creativity is to add a little bit of intention to explore this as a way to nourish not only your body but your energy body as well. It is also lovely to then share the food you make with another as you tune into the relational aspect of your water element. If you don't have another person around, you could share your meal with a pet or with the wild creatures outside your door. You could even consider leaving an offering for the nature spirits or the elementals that live all around you. If you don't have the time or ability to express yourself in an elaborate way, then at the very least you could take in other people's creativity by reading poetry or looking at art. Sometimes when I am wanting to dip into a pool of creative energy to jumpstart my own creative juices without having to do anything or go anywhere, I will look at art on Pinterest or Google. I get so much pleasure, satisfaction, and inspiration this way, and it is so easy to do!

Whatever you do, the objective is to allow your creativity to flow. Whether you can access this in abundance, in short gushing spurts, or even if it is just a trickle at first, notice how tapping into your creativity nourishes your second chakra when you do it with joy and playful curiosity.

Daily Affirmation

I am an inspired, creative being worthy of pleasure and play. I enjoy the process of exploring my creativity with curiosity, adoration and appreciation.

Daily Acknowledgment

What did you accomplish and/or how did you honor yourself today? What altar items did you choose? Document how you completed your daily soul-care ritual.

Daily Reflection & Journal Inquiry

What did you notice when working with your fire element today? Did you have any resistance around it? What felt nourishing to you?

Day Twelve: Earth Element

The earth element correlates to your root chakra, which is located at the base of your spine or perineal floor. It also expresses in your neck, bowels and knees. Your earth element deals with all things primal and foundational on the basest level. Fear and courage reside here. Earth rules your ability to feel grounded, supported, to have what you need for survival and to let go of what you don't need.

Today's Soul-Care Ritual/Prompt: Work with Stones for Grounding & Protection

Today's Soul-Care invitation is to work with stones for grounding, protection, and healing. You could sleep with them under your mattress, carry them in your pockets or even bury stones on your property if you want a more elaborate ritual.

Stones to balance your earth element

Some stones that work well for balancing your earth element could be red jasper, black obsidian, black tourmaline, hematite or tiger's eye.

How to work with stones to balance your earth element

Use one of the rocks mentioned above, or if you don't have any of these stones on hand, you could find one. Go take a walk outside your door and keep your eyes on the ground for a rock that calls out to you.

Find any rock that feels particularly earthy, grounding, comforting, calming or organizing to you energetically or physically. If you want to take this one step further, you could infuse this stone with your energy by carrying it in a pocket or placing it on your altar. Or you could sleep with it under your mattress or pillow.

Using stones for grounding and protection

Bury four stones in each of the four corners of your property with the intent to ground and protect the space where you live. You could say some words, create a ritual around this, or simply bury them and intend for that to be enough. Your intention is a powerful thing when combined with mindful action.

Daily Affirmation

I am safe, grounded, protected and whole. I have all that I need and I feel supported by the earth abundantly.

Daily Acknowledgment

What did you accomplish and/or how did you honor yourself today? What altar items did you choose? Document how you completed your daily soul-care ritual.

Daily Reflection & Journal Inquiry

What did you notice when working with your earth element today? Did you have any resistance around it? What felt nourishing to you?

Weekend Reflections

You are invited to go with the flow of your weekend and take time off from the challenge or use this time to catch up. To keep up your momentum, you may choose an element that needs more support or attention. Use the prompts below to tune into which element felt really good, and which one felt not so good.

Weekend Inquiry & Journal Prompts

What did you notice when working with all of your elements throughout the week? Did you feel or experience anything different or out of the ordinary, such as synchronicities or a new awareness?

Was there one element that you had resistance to more than the others? What about it was uncomfortable? Is there anything that you feel called to do to honor that or continue to work with it? What would it take for you to come into greater balance with this element energetically?

Was there one element that felt better than the others? What felt good about it? What happened or what did you notice in your body or life as a result of you tuning into this element?

How could you call on this element more to enhance your life and energy?

What is one thing you will do this weekend to honor your Soul-Care journey?

CHAPTER TEN: WEEK THREE

Day Fifteen: Ether Element

The ether element correlates to the throat chakra and is the first of the higher vibrational chakras to be embodied as a physical element through sound and space. Ether is associated with the non-physical and our relationship to our spiritual origins and our higher knowing.

Today's Soul-Care Ritual/Prompt: Pay Attention to Signs & Symbols

One way to balance the ether element is to pay attention to the signs and symbols that spirit, God/ Goddess, your guides or the Universe is trying to give you. The part of our higher intelligence that is connected to source and the collective consciousness knows that all things are connected and we are all essentially at the center of the universe. Our dreams, daydreams, signs and synchronicities are always guiding us and communicating with our inner world through the outer world. Paying attention and honoring when these special moments occur, allows us to nurture our connection to our higher selves and receive the guidance we need to find proper alignment within our energy system and our life.

Your prompt for today is to notice the symbols that come to you and record them in this workbook or a journal. Explore what they mean to you. You could also begin by tuning in to your throat chakra and acknowledging the ways you are open to this higher form of communication. You can even ask for a sign or symbol to come into your awareness today to help you find more balance and harmony in your energy and life.

How to balance your ether element through paying attention to signs, symbols and visitations

Most of us have had the experience at some point of thinking of something and then suddenly seeing that thing all the time (such as a particular kind of car or flower). Even if we thought it was uncommon, suddenly it is everywhere!

The Universe communicates with you in exactly the same way. Once you start to pay attention, the signs are all around you. The more you look for them and take notice when they happen, the more synchronistic events occur. This means looking at the world as though everything is connected and noticing all the ways Spirit is trying to reach out to offer you guidance and support.

One way to remain aware of when these things occur and to explore what they mean to you, is to keep track by writing them down. When you keep track of the signs, symbols and synchronicities that come to you in a journal (or this workbook), you give the universe the signal that you are paying attention. You begin interacting more with what shows up and you are more likely to take action on what is shown to you. When it comes to interpreting the signs or animal visitations that you start noticing more and more, try to refrain from using other people's meaning or symbolism and endeavor to make your own.

All symbolism comes from internal knowing, whether that is someone else's or your own. If you really want to research what things mean to other people or get to know more about the universal meanings of things, try what I call "google divination". This basically just means using the internet to type in a word describing the event, symbolic synchronicity or animal you saw, for instance, and then see what jumps out at you. What do you feel called to click on? What resonates with an inner 'A-HA' feeling? Be willing to be surprised and pleasantly pleased as the world unfurls its magic at your feet.

Suggested Daily Affirmation

I am in constant communication with the divine and the world speaks to me everyday in magical, beautiful synchronicities. I am awake, aware, and one with everything.

Daily Acknowledgment

What did you accomplish and/or how did you honor yourself today? What altar items did you choose? Document how you completed your daily soul-care ritual.

Daily Reflection & Journal Inquiry

What did you notice when working with your fire element today? Did you have any resistance around it? What felt nourishing to you?

Day Sixteen: Air Element

The air element is related to your heart chakra, which is all about love and generosity, beauty and playful self-expression.

Today's Soul-Care Ritual/Prompt: Immerse Yourself In Beauty

Today's prompt is to immerse yourself in beauty by collecting flowers or giving yourself a bouquet.

How to balance your air element through collecting flowers

This may seem like a simple prompt, but the act of gathering and assembling flowers or other natural materials, the physical beauty, and symbolism can offer powerful healing and have a balancing effect on your heart chakra.

The first part of this is to give yourself permission to go outside and collect some flowers. Go out in nature- or your neighborhood and look for beauty where you may not otherwise notice it. You do not need to look for the kind of flowers you find in a grocery store or flower shop. Anything that looks beautiful to you and is up for grabs will do. (Note: do not steal your neighbor's flowers as this has the opposite effect on your air element literally)! Generosity is a great way to balance your air element, and this goes for being generous to yourself as well. If you can collect some plants or weeds or branches that look beautiful or spark your creativity, then go for it!

If you are unable to collect things from nature where you are, then you could also go to the store and buy yourself some flowers. The prompt would then be to build a bouquet by yourself as opposed to buying one premade if possible. Notice which flowers call to you. Take time to smell them, feel the energy of each one. Which appeals to you? This process of engaging your senses, choosing and assembling something beautiful, and then gifting it to yourself is all balancing for the heart chakra.

You might choose to put these on your altar or put them in the most visible place in your home where you spend the most time. Every time you see these flowers or smell them in the air think a loving thought about yourself. Allow the beauty they bring to be a mirror of your inner beauty. Feel worthy of this because you are!

Daily Affirmation

I am worthy of pleasure and play. I immerse myself in beauty and generosity both inside and out. I am love.

Daily Acknowledgment

What did you accomplish and/or how did you honor yourself today? What altar items did you choose? Document how you completed your daily soul-care ritual.

Daily Reflection & Journal Inquiry

What did you notice when working with your air element today? Did you have any resistance around it? What felt nourishing to you?

Day Seventeen: Fire Element

Your fire element resides in your solar plexus, thighs, eyes and forehead. Your fire element rules your ability to visualize the future you want to manifest and the will to discern what action to take so you can bring your ideas into physical form.

Today's Soul-Care Ritual/Prompt: The Archer/Manifestation Exercise

Today's soul-care prompt is one of my favorite Polarity Therapy energy exercises that I have adapted over time into a manifestation and visioning exercise as well. I call this exercise the archer because the movement is similar to using a bow and arrow.

By harnessing the potency of your will and directing conscious, focused thoughts through your gaze, you can see the target and manifest whatever you are calling in and ready to take action on, with power and clarity.

How to do the archer exercise

This exercise looks and feels similar to the warrior pose in yoga. If you know how to do the warrior pose, you can use it to fuel your fire element in a very similar way. To begin the archer, you will start by tuning in to your solar plexus chakra. Close your eyes, place your hands just above your diaphragm, take a deep breath, and feel your power center. Allow it to help inform you of an intention that you would like to call in. This could be something you want to do, make, create, or it could even be as simple as intending to balance your fire element or hone your ability to be decisive and empowered.

Once you know what you are focusing on mentally, you will start with both hands bent at the elbow meeting at your solar plexus. Slowly move your left hand out across your body, staring sharply down your middle finger the whole time in slow motion. The eyes direct your energy, and the middle finger is the elemental line for your solar plexus chakra. Staring down your left middle finger, extend your arm so that the right arm is still bent at the elbow like it is drawing back your bow, and your left is letting the arrow fly. As you release your imaginary arrow, focus on your intention, and imagine that you are calling in all the resources you need to make this happen. Whatever you need, it will come.

Slowly bring your left arm back to center, and as soon as your middle fingers touch, slowly extend your right arm so that you are now releasing your arrow to the right side while your left arm is steadily holding the bow. As you stare fiercely down your middle finger, imagine yourself accomplishing the task, achieving the goal, or creating the thing you are intending. See it, feel it, and know that it is possible. As you send your arrow of intention out into the universe, you are exercising your powerful creative abilities and calling on the universe to support you in your endeavor.

When to use this exercise

This is an excellent exercise to use if you are feeling indecisive, disempowered, disconnected from your essential self, or distracted and unable to focus. You can do this before you have to go to a meeting or have a difficult conversation, or you could use it to empower a project with greater ease and potency. The uses are limited only by your imagination. Just like you! Imagine it, feel it, embody it, and know that you can create with clarity and power.

Daily Affirmation

I am a powerful creator manifesting in total alignment with my highest self. I have all that I need and know exactly how to create from a clear, focused, empowered place inside myself.

Daily Acknowledgment

What did you accomplish and/or how did you honor yourself today? What altar items did you choose? Document how you completed your daily soul-care ritual.

Daily reflection & journal inquiry

What did you notice when working with your fire element today? Did you have any resistance around it? What felt nourishing to you?

Day Eighteen: Water Element

The water element correlates to your second chakra, which is the most receptive of all the elements. It is receptive in the sense that it is responsible for the parts of you that give and receive pleasure, experience childlike joy and playful abandon, creativity, connection and embodied intuition.

Today's Soul-Care Ritual/Prompt: The Body Pendulum

Working with your physical intuition can be very powerful for both clearing and enhancing your second chakra. One way to do this is to tap into your deeper intuitive senses by listening to your body's guidance. Today's exercise is called the body pendulum. This is related to applied kinesiology. You can use this method to check and balance any of your energy centers.

When we dive into the deep waters of the second chakra, we can feel our subconscious or inner guidance through our physical embodiment of the divine. We can access our inner knowing and empathic or kinesthetic intuitive abilities. It is very balancing for the water element to pay attention to the ways we receive guidance from our body and our empathic knowing. We can also increase or moderate these abilities in the most balanced way when we tend to our water element by bringing our loving attention there.

How to do the body pendulum

1. To begin, you will want to make sure you are adequately hydrated by drinking some water.
2. Come to a standing position with your knees and eyes soft.

3. Tune into your second chakra by placing your hands on your abdomen. Drop your awareness into your body. Notice how your second chakra feels, what images or colors you see, and if you feel comfortable or uncomfortable being

4. here with your body in this way. Just notice and honor whatever comes up.

5. Keeping one hand on your abdomen, move your other hand up to your heart and tune in to a feeling of gratitude and love. You can do this by thinking of someone or something you love dearly like a pet or a baby, or anything that feels pure and easy to connect to. By attuning to feelings of love and gratitude, you are elevating your energy, thereby

6. creating a more accessible line of communication between your body's highest wisdom and your interpreting mind.

7. Ask a simple yes or no question that you know the answer to then allow your body to rock either forward or backward. I usually ask something like, "is my name Amanda?" I know this is true, so my body will sway forward so that I am rocking up onto my toes.

8. Ask an easy question that you know isn't true, such as, "Is my name Bob?" Unless your name is Bob, you will feel yourself falling backward ever so gently.

Now that you have established a way to interpret Yes and No answers, you can use your body as a pendulum to ask anything that you need to know. I often use this to determine if I should take a certain supplement, eat certain foods, attend an event, and I have even used this method to choose paint colors!

Using the body pendulum to balance your energy

Do you need more water energy? Are you overly waterlogged and need something else? Ask your body to give you an image or inspiration of what that might be and test it with the body pendulum.

You can ask if there is anything you need to let go of- such as other people's energy, unhealthy attachments, boundaries you need to clean up within yourself or with another. You can visualize the color orange, imagine a beautiful waterfall cleansing your energy body, or imagine sending some energy from your heart to your abdomen. Infusing your second chakra with loving, healing intentions can be enough to shift things dramatically. After you do this, rate your water element again.

You are welcome to try this exercise with any or all of your energy centers as needed or to make other decisions that you are having a hard time with mentally. Your body is incredibly wise. It is a vessel for your highest knowing, and it's very healthy for your second chakra to trust what your gut is trying to tell you!

Daily Affirmation

I am a wise creator being, and I have all the answers within. I trust myself and honor my body's wisdom.

Daily Acknowledgment

What did you accomplish and/or how did you honor yourself today? What altar items did you choose? Document how you completed your daily soul-care ritual.

Daily Reflection & Journal Inquiry

What did you notice when working with your fire element today? Did you have any resistance around it? What felt nourishing to you?

Day Nineteen: Earth Element

The earth element is related to your root chakra, which is all about your connection to your physical wellbeing, your ability to be supported and feel safe in the world. Even though we are of the planet and exist in an abundant beautiful world, there are many times in life when we do not feel like this or cannot access it internally or externally. By intentionally connecting with nature (even with our imagination), we can help to nourish our earth element, which can restore our ability to be abundantly supported and rooted.

Today's Soul-Care Ritual/Prompt: Forest Bathing

Your root chakra is greatly nourished by connecting with the earth itself. For today's soul-care prompt, you are invited to connect with nature through forest bathing. If you are unable to go outside and connect with an actual forest for any reason, I have included other suggestions as to how you can do this at the bottom of this section.

What is Forest Bathing?

Shinrin-yoku is a term that means "taking in the forest atmosphere" or "forest bathing." Shinrin-yoku Forest Therapy was developed in Japan during the 1980s and has become a cornerstone of preventive health care and healing in Japanese medicine.

From 2004 to 2012 alone, Japanese officials spent about $4 million dollars studying the physiological and psychological effects of forest bathing. One professor in Tokyo measured the activity of natural human killer (NK) cells in the immune system before and after exposure to the woods. These cells provide rapid responses to viral-infected cells and respond to tumor formation and are associated with immune system health and cancer prevention. Studies have shown significant increases in NK cell activity in the week after a forest visit, and positive effects lasted up to a month. The conclusion?

Forest bathing is good for your health!

This is due in part to the phytoncides found in various essential oils of wood, plants, and some fruits and vegetables, which trees emit to protect themselves from germs and insects. Forest air doesn't just feel fresher and better, inhaling phytoncide seems actually to improve immune system function. In other studies, being in the forest has also been found to promote lower concentrations of cortisol, lower pulse rate, lower blood pressure, greater parasympathetic nerve activity, and lower sympathetic nerve activity than do city environments.

Many other studies have proven the immense benefits that being near trees have on our body, but forest medicine is good for both body and soul. It affects our whole being, as our subtle electromagnetic field is charged and cleared by being in nature and connecting with the earth.

How to Forest Bathe

Forest bathing is a simple process of being outside in the forest while doing... nothing else. Just being in nature without walking, talking, moving, running, counting steps, or thinking (to the best of one's ability). Connecting with the natural world and increasing your awareness of the subtle qualities that begin to wash over your senses, is forest bathing. It is cleansing, nourishing, and renewing on all levels. If you do not have a forest accessible, you can use this conscious awareness of the health of being near trees and find any tree near you. Even a small city tree will do. Sit with the tree, talk to the tree, touch the tree, engage all of your senses. If you can't find a tree, use a plant. If you don't have a plant, use your imagination. Even that is good for your health!

Daily Affirmation

I belong to the earth as the trees, plants and animals all do. I am nourished and healed by my connection with nature. The earth supports my body, mind and soul.

Daily Acknowledgment

What did you accomplish and/or how did you honor yourself today? What altar items did you choose? Document how you completed your daily soul-care ritual.

Daily Reflection & Journal Inquiry

What did you notice when working with your earth element today? Did you have any resistance around it? What felt nourishing to you?

Weekend Reflections

You are invited to go with the flow of your weekend and take time off from the challenge or use this time to catch up. To keep up your momentum, you may choose an element that needs more support or attention. Use the prompts below to tune into which element felt really good, and which one felt not so good.

Weekend Inquiry & Journal Prompts

What did you notice when working with all of your elements throughout the week? Did you feel or experience anything different or out of the ordinary, such as synchronicities or a new awareness?

Was there one element that you had resistance to more than the others? What about it was uncomfortable? Is there anything that you feel called to do to honor that or continue to work with it? What would it take for you to come into greater balance with this element energetically?

Was there one element that felt better than the others? What felt good about it? What happened or what did you notice in your body or life as a result of you tuning into this element?

How could you call on this element more to enhance your life and energy?

What is one thing you will do this weekend to honor your Soul-Care journey?

CHAPTER ELEVEN: WEEK FOUR

Day Twenty-Two: Ether Element

The ether element relates to the throat chakra, which is the doorway between this reality and the more etheric multidimensional versions of reality perceived by the upper chakras. When your ether element is in balance, you have a greater capacity to access these higher realms through your upper more spiritual chakras. You can access your intuition by opening the flow of communication between your conscious mind and your (third eye chakra) vision, and (crown chakra) higher knowing.

Today's Soul-Care Ritual/Prompt: Dream Seeding

For today's prompt I am sharing a very basic way to begin working with your dreams for intuitive guidance called Dream Seeding. You can use this to strengthen your communication with your higher guidance, spirit, or source, so that you can live in greater alignment physically, creatively, energetically and spiritually.

What does it mean to seed your dreams?

Dream seeding also known as Dream Incubation, is a term in DreamWork we use to describe a process of setting an intention to receive guidance, instruction, or to dream on a particular topic or go to a specific location. You write down your intention before you go to sleep and commit to paying attention to the dreams that come. You can begin by tuning in to your ether element and getting clear on a question you have for your life; about your energy, relationships, work, creativity, or anything you would like guidance around. Through DreamWork, you can receive inner guidance for your energy and your life.

How to seed your dreams for guidance

In order to seed your dreams, you will begin by writing down your question in a journal or inside this workbook. Ask your body, your highest wisdom, and your guides, ancestors, or whatever higher power you have a relationship with, to bring you a dream you can remember. Make sure to write these words as part of your request. If you are not sure what to ask, you could ask for your highest guidance to bring you whatever dream you need that will support you most on your journey right now. As soon as you wake up, record the dream that came to you even if it seems unrelated or fragmented. Often our dreams reveal their meaning after the fact. If you have a hard time remembering your dreams, try not to move when you first wake up. Often our body remembers when our brain forgets.

If you are interested in exploring more ways to work with your dreams, go to Elevationhive.com/soul-care-book for free resources including access to a free Dream Seeding foundations class. If you don't remember your dreams or only have short seemingly random dreams and want to learn more, then check out my blog post on how to increase your dream recall and work with dream fragments. Both of these resources are listed under Dream Seeding.

Dream seeding and other DreamWork practices have been the most powerful tools I have ever found for direct guidance, self-development, and healing. Definitely worth exploring if you are interested in developing your intuition and learning how to connect with your energy more deeply!

Daily Affirmation

I am supported by the Universe. I have an entire spiritual entourage looking out for me. It is my birthright to work with my intuition, dreams and higher knowing. I am open to receiving the guidance that is available to me.

Daily Acknowledgment

What did you accomplish and/or how did you honor yourself today? What altar items did you choose? Document how you completed your daily soul-care ritual.

Daily Reflection & Journal Inquiry

What did you notice when working with your ether element today? Did you have any resistance around it? What felt nourishing to you?

Day Twenty-Three: Air Element

In Polarity Therapy, the air element which relates to your heart chakra, can be balanced by working with the shoulders, chest or upper back and ankles. The air element flows around your body like a spiral current of energy, which travels East to West, side to side. This energy current is related to your heart chakra and your mental faculties. Often when the East-West current is either congested and stagnant or too wound up, we find it hard to settle, focus, meditate, or organize our thoughts.

Today's Soul-Care Ritual/Prompt: East-West Exercise

Today's soul-care prompt is to clear your heart chakra and mental plane by working with the East-West energy current. I will share a Polarity balancing exercise and a few other ways to connect with your heart chakra to assist in clearing energetic congestion, settling anxious cyclical thoughts, and balancing the East-West energy flow.

Before you attempt to make any shifts, we want to notice and honor where you are. You can tune into your heart chakra by closing your eyes, placing your hands on your chest on your heart area, and tuning in to notice how this area of your body and energy feels. If you could imagine a spiral of energy moving around you from side to side, what would it look or feel like? What is the quality of your experience as you tune in to this area? Does it feel rapid and anxious or constricted and unmoving? What emotions or sensations arise? Does it need more or less energy? Is it excessive or deficient? On a scale of 1-10 how balanced does this area feel?

How to do the East-West Energy Current Balance

Once you have established a general idea of how this area feels you will begin by bringing your arms up, bending them 90 degrees at your elbows like a saguaro cactus, as one of my colleagues likes to say. With your legs widely planted, gently begin to rotate at the hips breathing in through your nose and out through your mouth. Your arms will make a sweeping motion from side to side. I like to imagine that I am sweeping clean any mental debris that is clogging my energy field.

Slowly pick up speed and begin to breathe more vigorously. When you are ready you can begin to wind down your movements until you are still. Stand in place before you move and notice how your heart chakra feels. Rate from 1-10 again, so you can tell what has shifted.

A note about the East-West Exercise

If you do this for more than a minute, it can get exhausting, but if your air element is feeling stagnant or constricted, it can be highly beneficial to keep going long after it gets uncomfortable. I have personally experienced tremendous heart opening from doing this exercise vigorously for several minutes. It resulted in a spontaneous emotional release which allowed for healing and softening of my heart center in a profound way. I have also taught this exercise to hundreds of clients over the years and some have reported back that their chronic headaches went away, anxiety or nervousness was reduced, communication issues were resolved, and other spontaneous air related healings have occurred. These exercises seem simple but trust me when I say, they are super powerful.

A counterbalance to the East-West: The Integration Hug

If you are feeling unsettled, ungrounded or too airy, this next exercise can be very soothing. It is also nice to try as a follow up to the East-West. As one of the physical areas to balance the air element resides in the shoulders, you are invited to cross your arms, resting your hands on your shoulders as though you are giving yourself a hug. In Polarity Therapy, whenever we go through an emotional or energetic process, it is observed that an integration period is necessary. Often clients will begin to do this naturally by crossing their arms, legs, ankles, or folding their hands together. When we make these physical gestures, they is very integrating for the right and left hemispheres of the brain. This pattern imitates the two energy currents that crisscross up the body known as the caduceus.

While folding your arms across your chest hugging your shoulders, you can tune into your heart center and imagine that you are resourcing your body's ability to integrate your life, mental issues, emotions, or whatever causes your heart chakra to move out of balance. Imagine that you are hugging yourself as though you are your own dearest friend or beloved partner. This kind of gesture is incredibly healing and settling for the air element. You can stroke your shoulders, whisper sweet nothings to your own heart, and take a moment to receive some loving kindness from yourself to yourself.

If your heart could share a message with you in this moment, what would it have to say? What in your life might open or shift if you were to pay attention to your heart like this on a regular basis?

Daily Affirmation

My heart is open, balanced, strong and clear. I choose to live in harmony between my heart and mind. I respect, appreciate and honor myself exactly as I am.

Daily Acknowledgment

What did you accomplish and/or how did you honor yourself today? What altar items did you choose? Document how you completed your daily soul-care ritual.

Daily Reflection & Journal Inquiry

What did you notice when working with your air element today? Did you have any resistance around it? What felt nourishing to you?

Day Twenty-Four: Fire Element

Your fire element rules your solar plexus chakra which is a powerful, embodied, action oriented energy center associated with the color yellow like the sun. In Polarity Therapy there are three physical expressions that energy takes which in Sanskrit are called the three Gunas. These are sattvic, rajasic and tamasic. The sattvic expression is associated with air or ether. It is still and soft. The tamasic expression is associated with water or earth, which is deep, slow and penetrating. The rajasic expression is associated with fire, which involves faster more vigorous movements such as shaking or gyrating.

Today's Soul-Care Ritual/Prompt: Shake, Move, Dance & Get Rajasic

One of my favorite ways to balance the fire element is through rajasic movement. You're invited for today's soul-care prompt to explore this for yourself and notice how the simple act of moving your body can have a ripple effect on your life.

How to do rajasic movement

One way you can really get your fire element revved up is to put on some fast music and dance wildly. Jump, bounce, flail your arms and let yourself go with wild abandon. Be like Animal from Jim Henson's *Muppets*. Be like a whirling dervish. Make like you're in the movie *FlashDance* or *Footloose* and let your sweat fly. I love to put on African drumming music to accompany this, but you can try anything faster and percussive or whatever makes you move furiously. Do this to the degree that you are able-- modifying as necessary to accommodate your optimal activity level.

Engaging in rajasic movement is a great way to get your inner fire started if it is slow or flickering. If you want to empower a project, bring more energy to accomplish something you have been putting off, or feeling resistance to, this can be a great way to get your fire started. Conversely if you are suffering from too much fire and need to give it a safe contained way to burn itself down a little, you can give yourself permission to channel that energy through your movement. This is especially helpful if you have repressed anger or rage. Try jumping, shaking, yelling and giving yourself permission to MOVE THAT ENERGY OUT OF YOUR BODY. Better out than in, as the saying goes. Often when we are stagnant or stuck in our fire element, we have a hard time just hopping up into an exercise like this. If you read the above prompt and felt like crawling under your covers and taking a big fat nap, then you could try a different polarity exercise first or even instead of the rajasic movement.

The Ram Thigh Rub

This exercise involves using both sound and movement. The mantra for the solar plexus chakra is RAM. The three areas associated with the fire element in Polarity Therapy are the eyes, solar plexus and thighs. If you are able to come to a standing position that would be ideal, but if need be you can try it from sitting. While chanting the sound RAM, you will vigorously brush the palms of your hands down your thighs using a downward sweeping motion. Starting at the top of your thighs rub your palms down towards your knees. With each sweep down your thighs, you will chant RAM loudly. Do this at least ten times or more if you are able. I sometimes feel like I am trying to start a gas-powered lawn mower during this exercise.

The continuous RAM begins to sound like a motor getting started, and it can be fun to get guttural with it. The sweeping motion feels like it is in a way, related to pulling that cord connected to your inner engine. You may begin to build some heat in your hands, legs or body, especially if you are standing with your knees bent. This is good as you want to build heat and get the energy flowing. After doing this exercise try bouncing, shaking or dancing and see if you have less resistance to moving your energy rajasically.

Daily Affirmation

I am powerful, embodied, and capable of taking action in my life. My inner fire burns healthy and bright, and I know exactly how to tend to it. I let my inner light shine.

Daily Acknowledgment

What did you accomplish and/or how did you honor yourself today? What altar items did you choose? Document how you completed your daily soul-care ritual.

Daily reflection & journal inquiry

What did you notice when working with your fire element today? Did you have any resistance around it? What felt nourishing to you?

Day Twenty-Five: Water Element

Your water element rules your second chakra, which has to do with emotion, receptivity, and your physical intuition. If you are attuned to this aspect of your watery nature, you might be very empathic, which means you are the kind of person who picks up on other people's emotions or physical sensations easily. The water element is also responsible for your ability to let things go, and if it is out of balance, can result in addictive or codependent behaviors.

Today's Soul-Care Ritual/Prompt: Get Full of Yourself

Today's soul-care prompt is to bring your attention to your second chakra by tuning in and clearing the energy with your intention and loving attention. You are invited to take command over your body and energy by requesting any foreign energy to leave. You will also be learning how to get "full of yourself" in a humble yet powerful way.

Why is this practice important for empaths?

Oftentimes, we carry other people's energy or unknowingly pick up on other's emotions. If we are too energetically absorbent or sponge- like, then we will hold other people's energy in our body. The first practice to get clean and clear in your water element is to tune in and notice if there is foreign energy clogging your waterways. The second step is to fill your body with your own energy using a color, sound or intention. Being full of yourself is not a bad thing when we are talking about your big "S" Self (one with source) as opposed to the ego self.

What if you aren't picking up on anything?

The following exercise will help to balance your second chakra regardless of whether you think of yourself as empathic or not. If you feel like you have no problem whatsoever leaving other's emotions alone, you might even need to increase your receptivity.

How to tune in and clear the energy in your second chakra

To begin, you are invited to close your eyes and place your hands on your abdomen, sacrum (low back at the base of your spine), or one hand on each. Allow yourself to get into a relaxed state by taking a few deep breaths in and out. Ask your body if there is a color, shape, or image it wants to show you. Notice if you feel any emotions or sensations. The color orange represents the second chakra, but you might also see blue waves or a river or stream in your mind's eye. You might see something symbolic that is showing up to give you more information about what you need to bring to awareness to balance this energy center. If you don't see or feel anything at all, do not worry. Be willing to take your time and keep showing up for yourself, and more will come with time. In the beginning, it is good to know that just being here is healing, even if you don't sense a thing.

Ask your body if you have anything to let go of. Attachments, co-dependencies, or other people's energies. If so, state out loud, "I now release anything that isn't mine." Or you could say, "I now let go of any foreign energy or anything in my body that is not in my highest good or in the highest good of all."

You can visualize filling your second chakra with a beautiful orange light, or with whatever color feels most representative of you in this moment. *When we fill ourselves with our own energy, there isn't room to take on anyone else's.*

What to do if you feel like you are still carrying other people's energy in your body

Teaching empaths how to get a clean and stay sovereign is one of my specialties. This is due to the fact that I grew up as a sensitive, intuitive empath and had to learn (the hard way) how to use my sensitivities without getting overloaded. I had to learn how to tone it down when I needed to and turn it on high when it was appropriate and helpful in a way that benefitted me as well as others, as opposed to using it at my own expense.

The simplest way I know to clear your energy of other people's emotions or physical pain, is to ask it to leave. Tune in and command that anything that isn't yours must go. If you are sensitive, it might be good to do this on a regular basis. Other ways to cleanse your energy include taking a bath or shower, using sea salt on your head, wrists, feet or all over your body can also be clearing. Even being near water can help to clear your energy.

What to do if you are the opposite of empathic and need to increase your receptivity?

If you feel like your water element is more constricted then you might be holding your own emotions in too tightly or holding energetic boundaries that are too rigid to allow you to feel loved, accepted or connected to others. If you ever feel like people just don't get you, then it might mean that you aren't open to receiving the energy that is trying to find you and you may need to let more in, not less.

If this is the case, then you could replace the above statement with part of today's affirmation, which is, "I allow myself to give and receive energy abundantly in a balanced harmonious way." Imagine filling your second chakra with your own energy in whatever color feels most supportive for you. By tuning in to your second chakra with loving attention and awareness, you can balance your own energy, which could have a huge impact on your life. You may find that you are less prone to addictive behaviors, or that your personal boundaries improve. You might notice a more harmonious sexual expression as a result of this.

The water element deals with our ability to give and receive energy, pleasure, and tosense into the more subtle energies that exist on the physical plane. It can be helpful to do this exercise on a regular basis if these are trouble areas for you whether you feel excess or deficient. We are ever-changing beings, so you could potentially find yourself in either category on any given day.

Daily Affirmation

I allow myself to give and receive energy abundantly in a balanced harmonious way. I easily let go of anything that isn't in service of my highest good and the highest good of all. I am nourished, whole and complete as I am.

Daily Acknowledgment

What did you accomplish and/or how did you honor yourself today? What altar items did you choose? Document how you completed your daily soul-care ritual.

Daily Reflection & Journal Inquiry

What did you notice when working with your water element today? Did you have any resistance around it? What felt nourishing to you?

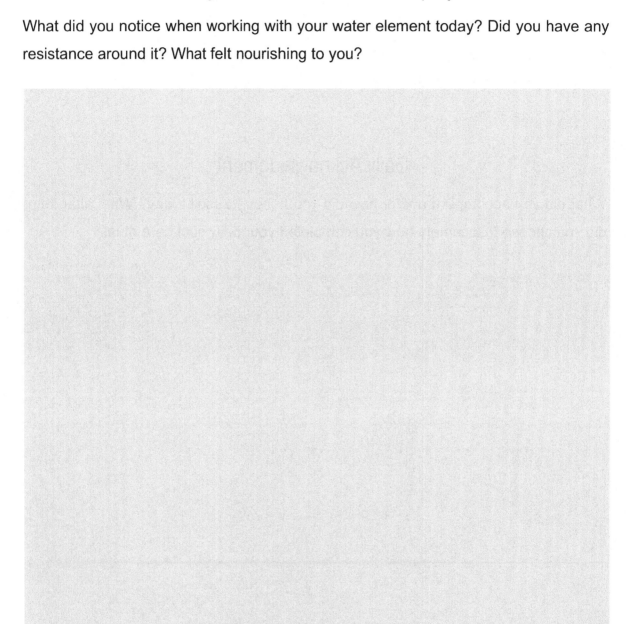

Day Twenty-Six: Earth Element

The earth element correlates to your root chakra, which is located at the pelvic floor or at the base of your spine. In Polarity Therapy the earth element can be balanced at the neck, colon, or knees. There are also minor chakras located at the bottoms of your feet. The earth element is associated with the sense of smell and the color red. Earth is the last of the elements to come into manifestation, so it is the lowest, slowest and densest vibrationally.

Today's Soul-Care Ritual/Prompt: The Wise Person of Old

Dr. Stone, the founding father of Polarity Therapy, used to say that if you only ever did one yoga pose out of all of them, the squat was the most superior for how it supports your ability to remain functional physically and energetically in your everyday life. I will be teaching you a squat variation from one of Dr. Stone's Polarity exercises, called the Wise Man of Old. I have changed the name of this exercise to the Wise Person of Old to honor all genders. We will be using essential oils, sound, and working with opening the hips through gentle polarity exercise. You are invited to add a gentle yoga pose called *Baddha Konasana* in Sanskrit, also known as the butterfly pose while we tune-in with a grounding visualization. Alternatively, you are invited to sit cross legged for this.

How to balance your earth element with essential oils

Essential oils have many powerful healing benefits other than just smelling amazing. They can cross the blood brain barrier through your skin providing powerful immune boosting support. They also offer mental, emotional benefits as they can travel from your olfactory nerves to the amygdala, which is the emotional center of the brain.

The essential oils I recommend for earth balancing are Frankincense, Vetiver, Black Spruce, Pine, Patchouli or you could try a blend. My favorite blend is Grounding by Young Living. I recommend using high quality essential oils such as Young Living brand if you are able. They might be more expensive than some other brands, but the quality and integrity of the sourcing of the oils is worth it in my opinion! But as long as the oils you are using do not have synthetic ingredients, you should get some therapeutic benefits.

You can place the oils on the back of your neck, on your low belly where your colon resides, the backs of your knees or bottoms of your feet. These are the areas that will be balancing for the earth element.

How to balance your earth element with gentle polarity exercises

One way to balance the earth element is through gentle movement. You can further connect to your root chakra by doing these exercises on the floor, with slow postures that open the pelvic floor and hips. To begin you will come into a squat or supported squat using a bolster, blankets, pillows, yoga blocks, a stack of books or whatever you have on hand to prop under your heels. You can lean your back against a wall for balance. Some bodies come into this posture easily, and some do not. There is no shame in being inflexible. I have practiced Ashtanga yoga almost every day for more than ten years, and I still cannot do a full squat with my heels on the floor! So, take it from me, there is no shame in using props to support your body.

How to do the Wise Person of Old

Once you are in a squatting position that works for you, fold your fingers together placing your thumbs on the inside of the ridge of your nose at the upper corner of your eye sockets. Lean your head into your hands putting the weight of your head into your thumbs and make a low OM sound.

This low toning opens the pelvic floor and harmonizes the root chakra. It is very relaxing and centering.

How to do a sitting posture with a grounding visualization

If you would like to try another posture, you can sit in *Baddha Konasana* also known as butterfly pose. Sitting on your bottom on the floor with your spine straight, bring your feet together, so your knees are resting towards the floor. Eventually the bottoms of both feet will be touching, or opening like a book. If you need pillows on either side under your knees to prop them up, that is absolutely fine. Find the posture that feels best for you. You could also come into a cross legged or lotus posture.

From here you can visualize your root chakra opening up to the earth, your spine growing into the ground like roots so you can exchange energy with the earth. Let go of anything you don't need and draw the healing nourishing earth energy up through your root chakra into your body. You can hum the sound OM in a low tone several times here if you would like.

Daily Affirmation

I surrender and open to the earth in sacred reciprocity. I give up anything I no longer need to be transmuted and receive the nourishment and support I need. I am safe, grounded and centered.

Daily Acknowledgment

What did you accomplish and/or how did you honor yourself today? What altar items did you choose? Document how you completed your daily soul-care ritual.

Daily Reflection & Journal Inquiry

What did you notice when working with your earth element today? Did you have any resistance around it? What felt nourishing to you?

Weekend Reflections

You are invited to go with the flow of your weekend and take time off from the challenge or use this time to catch up. To keep up your momentum, you may choose an element that needs more support or attention. Use the prompts below to tune into which element felt really good, and which one felt not so good.

Weekend Inquiry & Journal Prompts

What did you notice when working with all of your elements throughout the week? Did you feel or experience anything different or out of the ordinary, such as synchronicities or a new awareness?

Was there one element that you had resistance to more than the others? What about it was uncomfortable? Is there anything that you feel called to do to honor that or continue to work with it? What would it take for you to come into greater balance with this element energetically?

Was there one element that felt better than the others? What felt good about it? What happened or what did you notice in your body or life as a result of you tuning into this element? How could you call on this element more to enhance your life and energy?

How could you call on this element more to enhance your life and energy?

What is one thing you will do this weekend to honor your Soul-Care journey?

CHAPTER TWELVE: WEEK FIVE

Day Twenty-Nine: Ether Element

The ether element correlates to the throat chakra, which rules our self-expression and higher forms of communication. The most etheric form of anything becoming manifest in physical form is when it is spoken. Our words are a way to manifest, to give energy form even though it is still intangible. Ether loves spaciousness, silence, clear self-expression, listening and being listened to. In Polarity therapy, ether can be balanced in the body through the throat, jaw or TMJ specifically, any of the joints in the body, as well as all body cavities.

Today's Soul-Care Ritual/Prompt: Sound Healing

One of the best ways to open the throat chakra is through sound. Speaking our truth, repeating a mantra, chanting seed sounds, singing kirtan, or even partaking in karaoke or singing in the shower can activate and nurture our throat chakra. Sound moves energy, heals, opens, and clears energy blockages.

Sometimes when we feel like we need to cry but hold it in, we get "choked up." The emotion associated with ether is grief. Often when we are not fully expressing our emotions, allowing our story to be told or our pain to be witnessed, grief turns inward, and we can end up feeling constriction in our bodies or our lives.

How to balance the throat chakra with sound healing

The only difference between singing in the shower and balancing your ether element with song is intention. Even if you are unaware that you're affecting your throat chakra while singing, it will still be supportive. But when you sing or chant or make organic sounds with the express intent of opening your throat chakra, the healing benefits are greatly amplified. This is because consciousness also moves energy.

If you begin by tuning in to your ether element by bringing your awareness to your throat, you can imagine filling it with the color blue. Imagine all the space that exists inside your body. Then imagine all the space around your body. This is your sacred space. How much would you like to take up? If it feels supportive you can imagine a bubble, surrounding you. How much space does your bubble need? Expand it as far out as you want. Draw it in close and see how that feels. Then find the perfect most comfortable amount for you.

Tune into your body and energy and from this place of connection to yourself and your truth, invite any sound at all to come forth. It could be the strangest howl, squeak or a song you love to sing more than anything. It could be soft and shy or sharp, shrill, or guttural. Give yourself permission to make any sound that wants to move through you. Ask your ether element to let it out. Let it out!

If this is uncomfortable or you are lacking privacy, you could try going into a car and driving far away from people. Even blasting the radio and singing along at the top of your lungs will do.

If tears come, allow yourself to be in gratitude for the infinite intelligence of your body and energy. Whether you end up howling at the moon, laughing, crying or squealing hysterically, be willing to see your sounding as medicinal. After you have let your ether element express, see if there is a tone that feels comforting, healing, helpful, centering. It could be a low om or a high-pitched ooooohhhh. End with something calming and honor yourself for your courage, silliness, for freeing your spirit's greatness as you traverse this human experience that gives us the ability to make sound at all. What a gift it is to be manifest.

Daily Affirmation

I speak my truth and share my voice. I am spacious, worthy, safe and holy. It is my divine right to express myself fully.

Daily Acknowledgment

What did you accomplish and/or how did you honor yourself today? What altar items did you choose? Document how you completed your daily soul-care ritual.

Daily Reflection & Journal Inquiry

What did you notice when working with your ether element today? Did you have any resistance around it? What felt nourishing to you?

Day Thirty Air Element

The air element correlates to the heart chakra. Each of the elements has positive and negative emotional attributes. For the air element, the positive pole is unconditional love and generosity. The negative pole is greed or envy. When our heart chakra is open and flowing, we have limitless love to give to ourselves or others. When there are conditions to that love, or when we feel unable to let the good vibes flow, there could be unresolved hurt, feelings of unworthiness, or of not having or being enough.

Today's Soul-Care Ritual/Prompt: Practice Forgiveness

For today's soul-care prompt you are invited to practice forgiveness by writing a forgiveness letter. *To yourself.* This could be short and sweet, such as one sentence you write on a piece of paper and place on your altar, or it could be something you sit down and put some time into.

Why write a forgiveness letter to yourself?

We can hold onto grudges against others that will weigh on our heart, but usually we are aware of these. We usually know when we judge other people or when we feel hurt by them, and if we are doing our "work" then we know the importance of finding our way to healing around our challenges with others. But one of the less obvious and even more common (and insidious) ways the heart chakra gets out of whack is from holding on to uncomfortable thoughts, beliefs or emotions about ourselves.

Often these are feelings of resentment, envy, self-doubt or scrutiny. We can be perfectionistic and hard on ourselves, holding onto grudges we would never hold against someone else.

Have you ever said or done something you regret and then replayed the event over and over in your head? These things might seem inconsequential or too uncomfortable to look directly at, but in this exercise, you don't have to. You don't have to rehash old hurts or venture back into past traumas, mistakes, or broken-hearted moments. The only person you need to forgive is yourself. Right here and now in the present moment.

How to write a forgiveness letter for air element balancing

Depending on how much time you have to devote to this, you could choose to go about it in a couple of different ways.

1. Short and sweet

Write down today's affirmation on a piece of paper:

I am a sacred being worthy of love. I now release anything that does not serve me. I love and forgive myself completely.

You can place this on your altar. You could also speak this affirmation out loud to yourself while looking in the mirror.

2. The forgiveness letter (free-write)

If you have a little more time to devote to this practice, you could tune into your heart center and close your eyes. Ask your heart chakra if there is anything that is in the way of your fullest expression. Is there anything you need to release or let go of? If you are able to do a little freewriting or journaling around this, you might be surprised at what comes up. You could try using one or all of the following prompts to create a forgiveness letter to yourself:

> I am sorry for...
> I wish I didn't feel bad about myself for...
> What I would like to feel about myself is...

I forgive myself for…

I love myself for...

My advice for you in this process is to not get too caught up in your brain about it. Remember the heart rules the mind, and when out of balance, we can get stuck there indefinitely! So rather than thinking too hard, try letting yourself free-write your way there. This means that you will start writing, and don't stop until you are done-- even if nothing but gibberish comes out. Just keep writing. The good news about this letter is no one else is going to read it. You don't have to spell things correctly or edit it into a beautiful poem (although it could end up as one).

This is for you and you alone. The purpose of this letter is to support your heart chakra by clearing any unnecessary residue that may be lurking there. It's about bringing to consciousness the ways you might be judging yourself too harshly. Or judging yourself at all. This is for you to practice loving kindness, compassion and adoration toward yourself.

Once you have completed the letter, you can do whatever you want with it. Frame it and read it every day...

Burn it tomorrow.

Put it on your altar.

Put it under your pillow while you sleep and ask for dream guidance around it.

There is no wrong way to go about this. If you want to follow it up with a surefire way to strengthen your self-love muscles, go watch a funny movie or a standup comedian or try some laughter yoga. Nothing uplifts and clears the air element better than laughter.

Daily Affirmation

I am a sacred being worthy of love. I now release anything that does not serve me. With love, I forgive myself completely.

Daily Acknowledgment

What did you accomplish and/or how did you honor yourself today? What altar items did you choose? Document how you completed your daily soul-care ritual.

Daily Reflection & Journal Inquiry

What did you notice when working with your air element today? Did you have any resistance around it? What felt nourishing to you?

Day Thirty-One: Fire Element

Your fire element rules your third chakra located at your solar plexus and just below your diaphragm. It rules the part of your physiology that begins the digestive process by breaking down your food (whereas the earth element rules the eliminative aspect of digestion). Your fire element is also responsible for helping you process and digest the experiences and energy of life.

Today's Soul-Care Ritual/Prompt: Burning Ritual

For today's prompt, you are invited to assist and enhance the digestive and transformational aspects of your fire element with a burning ritual.

How to do a burning ritual to help balance your fire element

First, you will want to tune in to your fire element at your solar plexus chakra. Notice what images, emotions or sensations might be there. Does it feel strong or weak? Does it need to be ignited, rekindled, tended or does your flame need to be fanned? Do you feel overheated, irritated or inflamed?

The first step is to acknowledge and honor it as it is. Honor that it is working its hardest to process the energy of your life, and sometimes we need more fuel than we have access to in order to do this efficiently, or we need less gas poured on our wounds. Regardless of whether your fire feels excessive or deficient today, the next step is to do a little ritual to ignite and support the digestive transformative power of your fire.

To begin, you will want to gather a pen and paper, a candle and fire-proof bowl, or if you have access to a fire pit outdoors, you are welcome to go all out. As you tune-in to your fire element, identify one thing you would like to either call in or get rid of.

Is there a situation you want immediate healing around? Are there old, festering, angry feelings that you would like to be done with? Or perhaps as you are listening to your fire element, you are realizing that you need to put less energy toward a situation or person, and you would like to call your energy back. Or maybe you want to call in more decisiveness or some of your personal power, so you can take inspired action or fall in love with your life in a new way.

Whatever it is you want to transform you will write it down on the paper and fold it up. Before you burn it, tune into your solar plexus chakra and ask yourself how you feel about this issue on a scale of 1-10. I know the arbitrary numbers keep coming back but trust me- it is worth it to be able to measure how you feel before and after you burn the shit out of that piece of paper!

The next step is to call in your healing guides, ancestors, allies, spirit helpers, angels or the God/ Goddess of your heart, and call in the spirit of the fire element itself. Ask the spirit of fire to help you transform the energy around this issue. Even if you are not sure whether you believe in such things, ask anyway because it is good form and a respectful way to be.

Once you have connected with Fire, you are welcome to burn your paper. You may want to make sound, laugh, cry, bang a drum, jump up and down, or simply sit still and gaze into the flame intently. Do whatever you need to do to feel complete. Release your guides, safely extinguish your fire and know that the deed is done!

Now that you are done you can rate how you feel and know that the transformative process has already begun. If you are unable to burn something at this time, you can at the very least light a candle and use your intention and imagination. Ask Fire to assist you. It is happy to help!

A note about Fire's quick transformative powers

Many years ago, I worked with some *Ayani* shamanic practitioners who studied the ancient traditions of Peru. They were very much about ceremony and making bundles

And offerings called *Despachos* in a traditional way. They told me that if I ever wanted to transform something in my life slowly, that I should wrap my request in a bundle and bury it in the earth. The earth is the great transmutator and knows how to break things down. But the earth is slow. It might take years for your request to be transmuted by the earth completely. If you want to transform something quickly, they said, use fire. Fire will take something significant and dense and turn it to ashes in no time at all.

So, consider this when you want to invoke the elements. If you are ready to break something down and get a process going, fire is your ally. If on the other hand, you want to let something go in a slower, gentler way, then consider an earth ritual instead. You can use the same exact format I shared with you here, but instead of burning your paper you can bury it. I have done this with offerings both traditional and nontraditional such as chocolate, herbs, flowers or whatever feels most appropriate to you. Listen to the earth and allow her to inform you of a proper offering.

Daily Affirmation

Fire is my ally. It helps me process and digest my experiences fully and efficiently. I give up what I no longer need to be transformed instantaneously. I am free.

Daily Acknowledgment

What did you accomplish and/or how did you honor yourself today? What altar items did you choose? Document how you completed your daily soul-care ritual.

Daily Reflection & Journal Inquiry

What did you notice when working with your fire element today? Did you have any resistance around it? What felt nourishing to you?

Day Thirty-Two: Water Element

The water element correlates to the second chakra, which houses our ability to give and receive pleasure, go with the flow, be spontaneous, playful and connected to our deepest, intuitive, most authentic selves.

Today's Soul-Care Ritual/Prompt: Sacred Play

Today's soul-care prompt is to tap into the pure wise innocence of our inner child, so we can free up energy in our second chakra and engage in some sacred play. The water element is associated with inner child work. In each of us, there is an inner child who is connected to their body and dreams in a pure way.

At one point you knew who you were and what you loved. You even knew why you were here. You were clear, inspired and connected to your soul's deepest, truest purpose. Oftentimes, as we go through life, we get messages either directly or indirectly that we are not enough, or that our ideas are impractical or unrealistic. Shame for who we are, shame for how we look physically, and self-doubt are all learned qualities that come only *after* we encounter negativity. We don't start out believing we can't. We start out KNOWING that we can!

How to tap into your inner child

Before you run outside and start hula hooping, I want to invite you to tune into your second chakra and make connection with your inner child. Placing your hands on your abdomen, you are invited to close your eyes and bring your attention into your second chakra in your lower abdomen and sacral or low back area. Imagine that deep inside your pelvic bowl, there exists a younger childlike version of you. This part of you knows who you were before you came into this body, and they know who you will always be. This is the infinite all-knowing part of you that is innocent, authentic and in touch with your deepest truth. This is your wise inner child. The one who is joyful and free, unburdened by whatever challenges your soul signed up for this time around.

We almost always have a wounded inner child as well as a wise inner child. The wise one knows what the wounded one needs and is able to communicate with you what even your preverbal self possibly did not receive. It is good to acknowledge both of these versions of you if you encounter them. And it is possible that your wise inner child may have a message for you about how you could honor your wounded child today. You are welcome to receive whatever guidance they might have.

In addition, you could write a letter to your inner child. Or let your wise inner child write a letter to you-- through you. What do they want you to remember about yourself? What is it about your purpose, your pleasure, your play that would be most medicinal for you to revisit today? Was there something they weren't allowed to do when they were younger that you have the power now to give to them? Was there something that you loved more than anything that you haven't done in the longest time? Choose one action that really honors your inner child. It could be as simple as eating an ice cream cone, playing dress up, or going out and grabbing that hula hoop after all. Whatever it is your inner child tells you to do, it is good to honor it with some kind of action no matter how big or small.

Engage in Sacred Play

Sacred Play is any activity that brings you delight and puts you in touch with your most authentic essential self. It is a devotional act of love and respect. It is a kind of tending that disregards the social norms, your ideas of what is allowable, acceptable, reasonable, efficient, responsible, or anything else that your adult self normally expects. Sacred play is when you say yes to engaging in an activity with a conscious intent to love and honor yourself. Sometimes the idea of play evokes feelings of guilt or competitiveness or we might not feel like it is allowed. Even if we have creative or recreational outlets that provide a way for us to tap into this, it is not exactly the same. Sacred play could be something you do for five minutes, five hours or five days. But it is not something your adult self would normally think to do.

Alternatively, It could be more of a quality that you bring to any activity. If you normally ride your bike to commute and sometimes feel that playful inner child coming out, sacred play could look like a bike ride with no particular destination where your only purpose is to consciously connect with your inner child. Let your child drive the bike and see what happens.

You might suddenly go much faster, or perhaps you want to slow down and take in the scenery more. Maybe you get lost in the physical sensations of wind in your hair and forget about life for a minute. You might start weaving in between the lines, or jumping over large curbs, or letting go of the handlebars and waving your arms in the air. Sacred play is more about the how than the what. It is about the quality of your experience, the intent to nourish yourself with simple pleasures, and the freedom to indulge in creative spontaneity and curiosity. You might be amazed at how healing any simple act with this intention can be!

Daily Affirmation

My inner child is wise and free. I nourish myself lovingly. I am worthy of engaging in Sacred Play, and I do so joyfully.

Daily Acknowledgment

What did you accomplish and/or how did you honor yourself today? What altar items did you choose? Document how you completed your daily soul-care ritual.

Daily Reflection & Journal Inquiry

What did you notice when working with your water element today? Did you have any resistance around it? What felt nourishing to you?

Day Thirty-Three: Earth Element

The earth element is the densest of your energy centers because it is the last stop on the pathway to manifestation. Dr. Stone the creator of Polarity Therapy called this the involutionary or step-down process. This is the journey that all things go through starting with their conception in the energetic realm, to thought, expression, emotion, action, eventually coming into physical form. In order to involute or step down from spirit to matter, things must pass through each of the elements until they finally reach the earth plane. Once things go through their life cycle, they return to the earth to be transformed or transmuted. We all return to the earth eventually, only to shed our physical form and start the cycle over again. In this way, the earth element is the place of completion.

Today's Soul-Care Ritual/Prompt: Completion Ceremony

In honor of the completion of this 33-day journey through your elements and chakras, the prompt for today is to hold a ceremony to mark the end of this transformational experience. The earth element rules your sense of smell, and the taste associated with earth is sweet. Holding a sacred ceremony is one way you could honor the completion of this or any cycle. Celebrating and honoring yourself for completing any endeavor is a beautiful thing. Whenever we cross the threshold from one experience to another, it is good to acknowledge yourself and fully bring it to the earth. This completes the cycle of involution and marks the end of one thing and the beginning of another.

Today's prompt is to create your own ritual inspired by the Mayan tradition of the Sacred Cacao Ceremony. You may use this to celebrate and honor the completion of any event in your life going forward to bring closure, resolution, pay proper respect, and honor your growth and process.

About the Sacred Cacao Ceremony

First of all, cacao in its natural form is very different from regular store-bought chocolate and cacao taken ceremonially is a whole other thing as well. The sacred cacao ceremony comes from South America, rooted in the Mayan tradition. Cacao is a medicinal plant with both physical and spiritual benefits.

Traditionally, the cacao used for this kind of ritual is unsweetened and usually comes in a brick. Once it is broken up into chunks, it is heated in a pot with hot water. Things that are added to the cacao could be a sweetener of your choice such as honey or agave and spices such as cayenne, chili pepper, cardamom, cinnamon or vanilla. The process of preparing the cacao is slow and intentional as is the process of consuming it. Prayers and songs are sung into the chocolate as it is melting, infusing it with love and sacred intentions. When it is consumed in a sacred circle with others, there are more prayers, songs, and deep authentic sharing from the heart. Often this is followed by dancing. This is all done in a very intentional way. The space is cleared beforehand, and prayers and intentions are spoken. There are often grounding meditations offered, prayers of gratitude to the earth, the spirit of the cacao plant, and for the sacred moment you are in.

There are many ancient traditions around how to perform a proper cacao ceremony which are taught and passed down in a sacred way. The prompt for today is not to learn how to perform a traditional sacred cacao ceremony in the Mayan tradition. Rather you are invited to explore how you can use cacao to make your own sacred completion ritual.

How to create your own ritual inspired by the sacred cacao ceremony

If you are inspired to acquire or have on hand some pure unsweetened cacao and want to perform your own version of a sacred cacao ceremony, then great. But that is not required. You could instead partake in some (preferably high quality) drinking chocolate. If that is not available, then even a small chunk of delicious chocolate will do. You could also do this completion ritual without any chocolate using only your intention. The point here is to create a ceremonial environment to honor the completion of your soul-care journey (or any experience you would like to mark as complete).

1. Once you have acquired the cacao or chocolate of your choice, you will hold it in your hands and connect to your ether element. Visualize your throat center and invoke sacred space by tuning in to your body and inviting in your guides, ancestors, God/Goddess, Angels, Highest Self or whomever you feel connected to spiritually. Ask for the space to be infused, protected and supported by their presence.

2. Drop your awareness into your heart center and allow yourself to feel gratitude for all that you have explored throughout this 33-days or however long it has taken and in whatever roundabout way you got to this moment. Feel gratitude for your entire journey without judgment. Honor the spirit of the cacao--of the earth, and of the community that has gone through this journey with you, whether you know them or are connected with them or not. If you are here, then you have participated in a collective field of others exploring their energy system through this process, and even if you did it in total isolation, you were not alone on your journey. Allow yourself to feel a sense of belonging and community within the collective field of others who are doing their personal work with good intentions to heal and grow.

3. If you have a word, song, prayer or feel called to share anything at this moment you are welcome to. Regardless of whether you are gathering with others or doing this by yourself, you are invited to speak a word of gratitude out loud to honor yourself and your journey.

4. Bring your awareness into your solar plexus, your fire element. Notice what you

feel in this part of your body and energy. If there is any movement or gesture, song or expression that comes to you as a way to honor your process and experience, feel free to express yourself.

5. Bring your awareness into your water element, second chakra and feel the physical sensations, honor the joy, pleasure and creativity you have cultivated within yourself. Honor any emotions that are present. If you need to cry or laugh, feel free to honor any and all emotions as sacred. Be willing to let go of anything you no longer want to take forward with you. You are welcome to speak that into space. If there is anything you want to call in, you are welcome to claim that as well.

6. Bring your awareness to your root chakra, earth element. Allow yourself to be filled with gratitude for the completion of this process. You can honor anything and everything that you have seen to completion in this moment.

7. So often we complete things without taking the time to honor and celebrate them. It takes tremendous energy and staying power to see things all the way through a cycle. It is important to give yourself permission to slow down, acknowledge what you have done. Let go of any unmet expectations and fully receive the potency of your unique way of getting to this moment. All things must come to completion at some point. No matter how they turn out, it is important to honor your process, grieve the things you did not complete, and celebrate the things you did. Finish consuming your cacao and take your time being still. Perhaps you want to sit in meditation here or lie down. When you are ready you could get up and dance or move your body if you feel called.

8. End the ceremony with gratitude and blessings. Thank your guides and spiritual entourage for accompanying you. Release them from the space and return to yourself as though you are reborn and able to move out into your life with a new clarity and perspective. Anything is possible from here.

Daily Affirmation

I honor all that I have brought to completion and let go of the past, stepping completely into the present moment with gratitude for the earth that holds me. I celebrate and honor this blessed journey.

Daily Acknowledgment

What did you accomplish and/or how did you honor yourself today? What altar items did you choose? Document how you completed your daily soul-care ritual.

Daily Reflection & Journal Inquiry

What did you notice when working with your earth element today? Did you have any resistance around it? What felt nourishing to you?

Grand Reflections

Now that you have completed the 33-day Soul-Care challenge, you are invited to reflect on what has transpired for you. Perhaps you want to go back through the workbook and check out your original intention on day one. Note what has changed and what has shifted. What do you know now that you did not know at the beginning?

Final Inquiry & Journal Prompt

Was there one element that you consistently had resistance to more than the others throughout the challenge? What about it changed for you? Is there anything that you feel called to do to honor that? What would it take for you to come into greater balance with this element energetically? How have you already harmonized with it more?

Was there one element that consistently felt better than the others? What felt good about it? What happened, or what did you notice in your body or life as a result of tuning into this element? How could you call on this element more to enhance your life and energy?

What is (at least) one thing you will do from here on out in your life to honor your Soul-Care journey?

CHAPTER THIRTEEN: NEXT STEPS

Congratulations! You completed the 33-day soul-care challenge! Now what?

Now that you have made it through this workbook, regardless of how you went about it, you undoubtedly have learned more about your energy system and how to bring it into greater balance. You have learned the basics of how your chakras work and how to come into greater harmony energetically using color, sound, scent, stones, movement, dreamwork, ritual, and the simple act of tuning in.

You have learned how to tell when you have too much or not enough of a particular element, and you have become acquainted with how and where you tend to fall out of balance. Most likely you have made some subtle or even not-so-subtle shifts and experienced some transformations in your body, energy and life.

I sincerely hope that you feel awesome for all that you have accomplished! I recommend that you continue to use this book as a reference for working with your energy. You can go through them sequentially or return to the exercises that were most impactful for you at any time.

One of my favorite ways to use books like this (or any book for that matter) is to ask for divine guidance and open the book at random to see what exercise would be best for me in regards to a particular question or even out of general curiosity.

What Now?

You are invited to join our membership and/or check out our website to find out when the next live group movement is happening through the 33-day Soul-Care Challenge course and join us as many times as you wish.

You may also want to check out some of our other online courses and consider if you would like to go deeper with your elemental education through our Polarity Therapy training. Thank you so much for doing this important work of tending to your energy system. It is such an honor to be connecting with you through space and time and these words and exercises. I would love to know how this went for you and would be thrilled to connect with you to offer support in your continued growth through our other programs or classes.

If you haven't already, hop on the private Facebook group or reach out via email and let me know how these exercises worked for you, where you got stuck, how you moved through, and what shifted as a result. I would absolutely love to know. I honor your process and am deeply grateful to have been a part of it.

If you enjoyed this book, please leave a positive review on Amazon or send me an email to let me know! You may direct all questions, comments, requests for bulk orders, or teaching or speaking opportunities to Amandalux@Elevationhive.com

For more information, resources, support and inspiration visit:

ELEVATIONHIVE.COM

For reader exclusive resources go to:

Elevationhive.com/soul-care-book

Join the community & follow

Facebook: facebook.com/schoolofenergymedicine

Instagram: Instagram.com/elevationhive

Pinterest: Pinterest.com/schoolofenergymedicine

SECTION FOUR: QUICK REFERENCE GUIDE

Quick Reference Guide

This quick reference guide includes a list of the physical and mental/emotional attributes that correlate to each element or chakra. If you are curious about a certain issue, pain, affliction, or life challenge, you can check to see which element it falls under and which exercises could be supportive.

For example:

If you are experiencing eye troubles you will notice "eyes" listed under the fire element. You could pick one or several of the fire element exercises listed below, use the affirmations that go with that element, wear or surround yourself with the color associated (which is yellow), use the suggested stones or altar items or try any of the fire element inquiries. From engaging in these activities, you may learn more about the underlying energetic cause of your condition or it could potentially assist you in your recovery.

Medical Disclaimer

It would be out of integrity to make promises or suggest that doing these exercises alone will cure you. **Please seek medical attention whenever necessary.** Allopathic medicine has its place, and I recommend that you treat yourself from every angle you see fit. I would never tell anyone to "will" their symptoms away. I believe in the power of belief, and I have seen amazing things heal right before my eyes. But I have also seen the opposite occur due to stubborn neglect. Be open to receiving miracles but do not rely on them. Be discerning and get all the care you need.

A note about imbalances…

Blocks aren't always bad. Often when you hear people talk about chakras, you hear that "blocked" energy is bad, or that open chakras are better than closed ones. This is a simplistic idea; however, that disregards the intelligence of our energy system and the internal compensations we must make to safely navigate life. We are multifaceted beings with unique energetic metabolisms. We all process our experiences differently. What one person shrugs off as no big deal, can cause major trauma for another. Some experiences are digested quickly, and others linger for years.

As you contemplate what could be "out of balance" for you, it is good to do so with curiosity while suspending judgement whenever possible. What words jump out at you? What exercises seem compelling? Trust what you are drawn to and allow the solution to unfold as you explore.

Ether Element

The following is a list of physical areas and attributes associated with the ether element. Issues that affect these locations could potentially indicate a throat chakra/ether element imbalance.

Joint pain

Arthritis

Throat issues

Jaw, TMJ issues

Face or head issues in general

Quiet voice or losing the voice

Hearing loss

Ear infections

Laryngitis, polyps, or other afflictions of the vocal cords

Thyroid issues

Big toe or thumb issues

Anything affecting other body cavities or having to do with spaciousness or constriction in the body

The following list contains mental/emotional attributes that could indicate a potential ether element imbalance.

Feeling spaced out

Inability for using rational judgement

No Boundaries-too much freedom

Difficulty functioning on the Earth plane

Challenge putting ideas into creation

"Option Paralysis"

Close-mindedness

Inability to see "the bigger picture"

Feeling disconnected from Source or Higher self

Feeling trapped

Fears around self-expression (throat chakra)

Repression of emotional expression

Prolonged Grief

Inability to express creatively

Inability to speak one's truth

Overtalking or unable to talk

ETHER ELEMENT EXERCISES

Create an Intention Statement: Page 81

Make a Living Altar: Page 102

Pay Attention to Signs & Symbols: Page 126

Dream Seeding: Page 150

Sound Healing: Page 177

Air Element

The following is a list of physical areas and attributes associated with the air element. Issues that affect these locations could potentially indicate a heart chakra/air element imbalance.

Shoulder issues

Kidneys

Adrenals

Ankles

Lung or chest issues

Heart issues

Thymus gland

Skin

Nervous system

Feeling sluggish

Non-responsiveness or slow to respond physically

Feeling jittery

Underweight

Headaches or congestion in the brain

The following list contains mental/emotional attributes that could indicate a potential air element imbalance.

Feeling anxious or nervous

High strung

Quick to respond without thinking

Mental blocks or being overly mental

Jealousy, envy or Greed

Negative humor or joking (wittiness) at the expense of others

Overly social

Restless

Too linear and fixed in thinking-all or nothing mindset

Stuck in list making mode- not taking action

Blocked in ability to feel for others or overly giving

Bargaining

Ungrounded

Talks too much too fast

Inability to express thoughts in a linear way

Lost in thought unable to think straight

AIR ELEMENT EXERCISES

Breathwork: Page 87

Two-fold Somatic Process: Page 106

Immerse Yourself in Beauty: Page 130

East-West Exercise: Page 154

Practice Forgiveness: Page 181

Fire Element

The following is a list of physical areas and attributes associated with the fire element. Issues that affect these locations could potentially indicate a solar plexus chakra/fire element imbalance.

Forehead, eye or vision issues Jaw or TMJ issues

diaphragm/ solar plexus

Umbilicus

Thighs

Urine

Shaking or tremors

Headaches

Blood pressure issues

Heartburn or digestive issues to do with breaking down food

Rashes or red itchy hives

Fevers inflammation

The following list contains mental/emotional attributes that could indicate a potential fire element imbalance.

Inability to focus or being overly focused- myopic

Volatile temper

Resentment or deep-seated unexpressed anger

Low self-esteem/ inability to interact with others withdrawn

Indecisiveness

Inability to take action

Too spontaneous acting without thinking

Overly passionate or unable to connect with passion

Overpowering, too dominant

Disempowered, unable to stand in one's power

Overly defensive or unable to defend oneself

Too abrasive or brash

Starts things without being able to finish them

Takes on more work than one can handle- overly ambitious

Too much vigorous exercise, not enough balance with downtime

Unable to get started

Unable to perform physical activities or discomfort with being embodied or active

Too defensive of boundaries/ looking for a fight

Not able to take action to protect one's boundaries or stand up for oneself

FIRE ELEMENT EXERCISES

Water Element

The following is a list of physical areas and attributes associated with the water element. Issues that affect these locations could potentially indicate a sacral chakra/water element imbalance.

Sacrum

Low back or buttocks

Lower abdominal region

Breast area

Feet

Pelvic bowl

Testes/ Ovaries

Bladder

Tongue or sense of taste

Lymphatic system

Areas that produce bodily fluids such as - saliva, tears, sweat, or mucus

Swelling

Bloating

Sexual dysfunction

The following list contains mental/emotional attributes that could indicate a potential water element imbalance.

Sexual disorders

Overactive or under-active sex drive

Overly protective of others

Emotionally Detached/lack of empathy

Empath overload/lack of energetic boundaries or taking on other people's emotions

Emotional overwhelm

Feeling overly emotionally vulnerable

Overly attached to the past

Addictions especially to foods, drugs, pleasure

Codependency

Blocked intuition or inability to dream or trust bodies wisdom

Inability to cry or express emotion

Stuck creativity/unable to let go or trust in creative abilities

Gullible, easily coerced

Immaturity, all play no work

Overly serious- all work and no play

Rigid/unable to go with the flow

Too go-with-the-flow, irresponsible or easily swayed

Inner child issues (overly associated or dissociated)

WATER ELEMENT EXERCISES

Earth Element

The following is a list of physical areas and attributes associated with the earth element. Issues that affect these locations could potentially indicate a root chakra/earth element imbalance.

Neck

Colon

Low back

Knee issues

Pinky toe/ finger

Anything to do with the sense of smell or loss thereof

Bone or blood issues

Pain or dysfunction in the perineum

Foot or gait issues

IBS or constipation

Obesity or aversion to movement

The following list contains mental/emotional attributes that could indicate a potential earth element imbalance.

Feeling stuck and unmoving

Ungrounded

Feeling physically unsafe and insecure

Overly methodical and slow

Spacey and disconnected from reality

Overly cautious

Stubborn

Rigid

Too scientific or linear

Unable to manifest

Unable to bring things to completion

EARTH ELEMENT EXERCISES

Balance Your Poles: Page 96

Work with Stones for Grounding & Protection: Page 119

Forest Bathing: Page 143

The Wise Person of Old: Page 169

Completion Ceremony: Page 196

Made in the USA
Coppell, TX
12 July 2020

30895215R00125